CW00939520

10 STEPS
TO
ACHIEVING
YOUR
GOALS

Mark Hutchinson

© Copyright Mark Hutchinson 2017
ISBN: 978-1-5272-1591-7

Mark Hutchinson has asserted his right to be identified as the Author of this Work in accordance with the Copyright, Designs and Patents Act 1988.

All rights reserved. No part of this publication may be reproduced, stored in a retrieval system, or transmitted in any form or by any means, electronic, mechanical, photocopying, recording or otherwise, without the prior permission of the copyright owner.

A CIP catalogue record for this book is available from the British Library

Printed and bound in Great Britain by Book Printing UK
Remus House, Coltsfoot Drive, Peterborough, PE2 9BF

The information in this book has been compiled by way of general guidance in relation to the specific subjects addressed. The author and publishers disclaim, as far as the law allows, any liability arising directly or indirectly from the use, or misuse, of the information contained in this book.

Contents

1. Introduction
2. The Psychology of Goal Setting
3. The Ugly Truths of Goal Setting and Success
4. The 10 Steps to Goal Setting
5. Step 1: Set a Date
6. Step 2: Detail is Key
7. Step 3: Manageable Steps
8. Step 4: Identify Skills and Knowledge Required
9. Step 5: Identify Your Obstacles
10. Step 6: People to Associate With
11. Step 7: What Is in it for You and Why?
12. Step 8: What Are You Prepared to Give Up?
13. Step 9: Affirmations
14. Step 10: Visualisation
15. Reflection – the Vital Bonus Step
16. Core Values and Daily Goals
17. Ten Things I Want to Do, Be and Have
18. How to Create the Ultimate Vision Board
19. Summary

- About the Author
- Example Goal
- Goals Worksheets
- The Story of the Falcon and the Crow

1. Introduction

If you plan to drive from London to Scotland, what are the chances of there being no traffic, and of every traffic light being green the whole 500-mile journey? It's unlikely, right? You will need a plan, as well as a sat-nav or a map. You are likely to hit traffic, roadblocks, diversions and multiple red lights on your way. But this won't stop you from getting to your end destination. The journey to Scotland is very much like the journey to achieving your goals. If you're running a business and you need to adjust your product line, this may be your diversion. When sales are not as fast as you hope they will be, this is potentially your traffic. Achieving goals is all about perception – realising that most things are just road blocks and traffic, and they won't stop you from getting there in the end.

Hi, my name is Mark. I am twenty-six years old, a business owner and fulltime forex trader. Over the past six years I've been perfecting my formula on goal setting that has enabled me to write down my goals, using a strict process, and achieve them by keeping me focused, determined and on track. When I first started in business, my initial thought was 'how can I make the most money?' As I've grown, and branched into personal development and goal setting, my values and thought processes have changed. Now it's 'how can I run a business and create something that a customer is going to take the greatest amount of value from? How can I make the greatest impact in others' lives?' This is now my main purpose and it's led me to writing this book. This was when, how and why the idea for 'the 10 steps to achieving your goals' was born!

When I first came across goal setting I knew nothing. I researched, as many would, and most of the suggestions I found told me to 'write it down and create a goal board'. This may sound very familiar to you, and similar to what you've already done up until the present, but it misses out many of the pieces to the puzzle of goal setting that I'm now going to share with you in this book.

Scenario

Okay, so you're sitting there right now and you've identified one or more things you want for yourself in the future.

Perhaps it's a new car or your first house, that promotion you've been pushing for, or to start your own business. Perhaps it's the satisfaction of running 5 km and crossing the finish line. Whatever it is, you have something in mind, and you want it.

So how do we get these things to come to life? Well, the first thing is to stop 'wanting' these things and instead decide you're definitely going to get them. You do this by turning your wants into goals.

Here is where I'd like to start talking to you about the goal setting process. I'll take you through it step by step and discuss how to break down your goals, using the right language, to make them as efficient as possible, turning them into real goals!

What to expect from this book

You're new to goal setting, or have been setting goals for some time and feel as if you're stuck, or just don't know if the steps you're already taking are effective.

As you read this book you will find not only the 10 simple steps to follow when approaching each goal but also the most important part – the psychology and language you use when writing out your goals. You will also find examples of goals and exactly how I would have written them out, showing you the correct use of language to bring the goal closer to you psychologically.

By the end of this book you will feel not only confident in your ability to write down your goals efficiently but also a sense of empowerment that you now have the key to unlocking the genius that you already are and getting your subconscious brain to work.

Setting goals is incredibly important for progressing in life. The trouble is, how do you know you're setting the right kind of goals?

Most people make the common mistake of choosing goals based on what I call your 'surrounding culture'. Your surrounding culture is the web of beliefs, habits, practices and mythologies of society that tell you how you should live your life. It's your surrounding environment that tells you that:

• You should get that degree.
• You should work until you're sixty-five and then enjoy life.
• You should get a nine to five job.
• You should get married.
• You should have children.

These goals do not always serve your happiness; instead, they serve an ideology upheld by many cultures. It isn't your fault. You are just a product of circumstance, but it doesn't have to be that way. The important thing is that you have made a choice to read this book and be open-minded.

You must first be open-minded enough to be completely honest with yourself. The best way to choose goals that align with your happiness is to first ask yourself these three important questions.

1. What amazing experiences do you want to have in your life?
2. What will help you grow and become the person you want to be and the best version of yourself?
3. In what ways can you/do you want to give back?

These questions will help you cut through the clutter, the noise, and the confusion of traditional goal setting, and allow you to focus on goals that will serve your happiness. This is really important; I've fallen short before in spending too much time on goals I thought I wanted to achieve based purely on surroundings. You need to dig deep and find out what you really want rather than what you like the idea of doing. If you like the idea of something, you may get as far as

3

writing down the goal and maybe taking some action. But when you come to a hurdle, it's very likely you'll give up, feeling not only frustrated but pulling out your hair, asking yourself questions like 'why I am I giving up so easily?' It's because, unfortunately, the goal is not aligned to your highest values.

This is what frustrates people, as many haven't spent enough time thinking about what they truly want. Most people just think they know what they want. I want to make this point very clear, and I cannot stress enough how important it is to align your goals with your highest values, so as not to become disappointed and disheartened if you don't achieve set goals.

If you're trying to achieve a goal without first ridding your mind of limiting beliefs, then you're cheating yourself. First build a mindset congruent with success, and then get to work. Believing you can is the first step.

90% of people do not write down their goals!

Writing down your goals does a number of things for you:
• It makes you accountable
• It gives you focus
• It reinforces your commitment to them
• It helps you remember them
• It brings the goal closer psychologically

Have you ever gone to the supermarket without a shopping list? Not writing down your goals is like going to the supermarket without a list; it's likely you will forget something.

If you'd like to verify the importance of goals, ask the most successful person you know if they have ever written down goals.

Let's get started…

'If you are working on something that you really care about, you don't have to be pushed. The vision pulls you.'
- Steve Jobs

2. The Psychology of Goal Setting

When setting goals, it's important that you understand the psychology of this before you start writing them down. When I first came across this information I was shocked at how important language is. So I want to take you through some psychology. When it comes to new things and new information, it's crucial that you approach this with an open mind!

In this book we take a look at positive affirmations. For those of you learning what they are for the first time, here is an insight:

Positive affirmations

Using affirmations is a way of having a conscious control over your thoughts. Affirmations are powerful statements that you should tell yourself regularly in order to train your mind to think more positively. Each and every thought you have is an affirmation. Each and every thing you say is an affirmation. Every time you say something negative about yourself, you are affirming that to be the truth, and this will attract negativity and further negative thoughts. Using affirmations, you can train your brain to think in a more positive, motivational way. Affirmations serve as declarations of what you truly think of yourself and the world around you. For example: if you look at yourself in the mirror every day and pick faults in who you are, all you will ever do and all you will ever see are the faults. However, if you stand in front of the mirror and only focus on all the things you like about yourself, over time you will begin to see more of the positives. Your mind will naturally see a more positive perception of yourself, and of life in general. The idea of positive affirmations is to uplift and inspire you through the creation of self-affirming and self-empowering affirmations.

When you first start saying or writing down affirmations they may not be true. But with repetition, they sink into your subconscious mind and you really start to believe them. Eventually they become your reality; they become self-fulfilling prophecies and become true.

Over time they overwrite any limiting or negative belief you have about yourself or about not being able to do something. They replace negative beliefs with positive thoughts, which will instill confidence, self-belief, positivity, drive, ambition and much more.

It is much easier to see an example of positive affirmations for confidence.
- I am a naturally confident person
- I am confident when speaking in public
- I am confident and love meeting new people
- Confidence comes naturally to me

These affirmations are just a few examples of ones that you could use or tweak for yourself.

Someone who is shy or unconfident can repeat these affirmations by writing them down and then saying them out loud. I don't expect you to shout these affirmations out loud, making people think you're a crazy person, but when you're on your own in front of the mirror and you get your whole body involved, this can start the process of cementing these affirmations in your mind.

Using positive affirmations gives you back control of your mind and the information it receives. It puts you back in the driver's seat; you're the captain of your ship. You're in control and this helps you to let the positive thoughts become who you are and want to be. Physiology is so important when saying affirmations; it is simply getting your body involved. Have you ever seen someone that's passionate about a topic they're speaking about? You can see it's almost as if their whole body is communicating and it's not just them speaking the words. Think about Obama when he is addressing an audience; he captivates the room not only because of what he is saying but because his whole body expresses his passion about what he is saying. It is because he believes what he is saying with absolute certainty. Whether it be true or not, '*Whether you think you can or whether you think you can't, you are both usually right.*'

Here are some simple exercises that can help you start practising. The first is about writing down affirmations and the second involves getting your physiology participating.

Exercise One: Start by picking one affirmation of your choice. It could be anything, but here is my example:

- *I love myself and I am comfortable in my own skin.*

I want you to get a journal and write this line out ten times. Put the date at the top and sign your name at the bottom of the page.

Exercise Two: Say this same phrase in the mirror ten times every morning whilst smiling. Get your hands and body involved as if you mean it – as if you want to share something with the world and speak like you want to be heard. I know this might seem slightly crazy at first but the whole idea of this is to do something dramatic to get you out of your comfort zone. This will shock your body into taking action. This is one of my favourite techniques I learnt when studying the work of Anthony Robbins. This truly was a game changer for me, as it advanced me into becoming the person I am now. Not only does it work for confidence, but it has worked in many aspects of my life. For example, as well as making me more confident I also used it for business and capital growth. '*I attract an abundance of wealth into my life*' is one particular affirmation that I have been using for a long time. It has kept me motivated throughout business projects and entrepreneurial ventures, instilling belief in myself that this is what I will achieve.

I want to introduce and explain a statement that sounds positive but has something to it that could be damaging.

> Example: Shaun is writing down his goals and affirmations and he writes '*I will never give up on my dreams*'. This may appear as a positive thing but let's take another look at the sentence.
>
> I will never give up on my dreams.
> I will never give up on my dreams.
> I will never give up on my dreams.
> I will never give up on my dreams.
> I will never give up on my dreams.

Now let's look back at our initial example...
I will **never** give up on my dreams.

The brain may often ignore the negative and that is exactly why this 'positive statement' can actually work against you. If I told you '**Don't** think about a black cat' you would naturally start to picture a black cat... now why is that? Let me explain.

Imagine a three-year-old toddler is told 'Do **not** push that button'. It is more than likely that he goes and pushes the button, regardless of the parent telling him to do the opposite.

As the toddler's brain is ignoring the word '**not**', he is hearing 'Do push that button', leaving the parents once again frustrated as to why their child will not respond to this command in the way that they want.

I will **never** give up on my dreams.
I will **never** give up on my dreams.
I will **never** give up on my dreams.
I will **never** give up on my dreams.
I will **never** give up on my dreams.

Now we can see, by looking at this affirmation in a different light, that all the brain may hear is:

I will give up on my dreams.

Let's say Shaun writes this down as a reminder in his journal every day five to ten times, reading it back to himself in his head and also reading it out loud. He almost has a consistent encouragement to give up on his dreams! I found this type of psychology fascinating, as speaking to successful people made me realise many already know this secret.

I had heard about people making this 1% change in their life and achieving a tenfold success. But I was curious to find out how or why, and I began questioning many of them about these small changes that were making significant impacts on their lives.

The story of Acer and Apollo comes to mind, a story that I came across in the past during my sales days. Acer and Apollo were two race horses that went head to head with each other in a race for the title. The first prize was £100,000 per race, with the second prize being £10,000. Of the ten races, Apollo won them all. His owners walked away with £1,000,000 and the horse in second place, Acer, earned only £100,000. The difference between the winner and second place for all races was the matter of half an inch: a photo finish. Yet such a small 1% difference made ten times more money!

This just goes to show that success is not always down to a crazy difference of results. It can be a small change that makes such a big difference.

Something as simple as changing a few words is paramount to your success when writing out goals, but is even more important to psychologically bring the goal closer to you.

Let's re-arrange that earlier sentence into something more positive than the negative self-sabotage affirmation.

I persist until I succeed.

So now we have the psychology underway we can begin looking at the steps in more detail.

'The pessimist sees difficulty in every opportunity, the optimist sees the opportunity in every difficulty'
-Winston Churchill

3. The Ugly Truths of Goal Setting and Success

Not everyone will support you

One thing that I had to understand very quickly is that not everyone will support you, even if they think your business idea or goal is amazing. I personally spent way too much time questioning why my friends weren't supporting me and buying my product or promoting it to other people. At first I took it very personally, and that's okay, but you need to realise that it's not because your friends are horrible people; a big part of their reaction is that they would love to do what you're doing, but feel like they can't take the sort of risks you are taking. It's important to remember that they don't hate you or your idea, they hate themselves as you may be a reflection of what they strive to be. The biggest tip I can give you is to keep friends and business as separate as possible; rely only on yourself and keep pushing – you have nothing to prove to anyone but yourself.

You will be sacrificing something else

When you set a goal, at first it's very easy to think that you can achieve everything you want now that it's written down. But writing down the goal simply isn't enough. Sitting and just watching TV, hanging out with friends all the time and always being available should now be a thing of the past – maybe not permanently, but definitely temporarily. You will have to sacrifice your current 'free time' to actually work towards these goals; they won't work on themselves. I myself have learned that going out with my friends every weekend and getting a full night's sleep every night will not help me to achieve my goals as quickly as I would like. I have had to sacrifice events and also work through the night because without hard work you will get nowhere. Goal setting is just the tool to help you focus and empower yourself to work on the goals, but the hard work comes from you. Achieving goals is not easy! It is proven that as humans we feel a deeper sense of fulfilment when achieving a goal after having sacrificed to get there. If we could plod along achieving goals and have no change in lifestyle it would be too easy and everyone would achieve goals, but this certainly isn't the case.

'Nothing in the world is worth having or worth doing unless it means effort, pain, difficulty... I have never in my life envied a human being who led an easy life. I have envied a great many people who led difficult lives and led them well.' - Theodore Roosevelt

S.M.A.R.T Goals

It is a very common thing when you are researching goal setting to come across smart goals. In my opinion, although this is recognised, it can also be detrimental to your growth depending on how you view the steps. Before anyone wants to bite my head off because you've used this method, allow me to explain why... Forbes Magazine has backed this argument as one step that can be damaging when setting goals.

The idea of this technique is the goals need to be S.M.A.R.T.
- Specific
- Measurable
- Attainable
- Realistic
- Time bound

This is the common phrase you'll hear when setting goals and I agree with all but one to a cartoon degree.

Realistic: From my broking days in the city, I quickly learned that the word itself is one of the most self-sabotaging things you can say when it comes to limiting beliefs. To have that as one of your values in achieving serious goals will leave you with nothing but frustration.

Stop and think about that word for a minute and ask yourself: 'Who do you know, whether they be in the public eye or not, who has achieved something great and initially thought it was unrealistic?' If they had thought this, they would never have started.

The idea of realistic is subjective; each person will have a different idea as to what they can realistically achieve. However, the word realistic in itself could limit your belief in yourself. Elon Musk may have had people tell him it was unrealistic to start an electrical car brand that would make people look at the motoring industry in a completely different way. However, to him, he saw it as within his capability. He may not have known he would get as far as he has with Tesla but he knew that, in reality, almost nothing is unrealistic.

In the 1950s, most people believed that it was impossible to run a mile in under four minutes. One man did not; his name was Roger Banister. In 1954, Roger Banister broke the four-minute barrier with a world record time of three minutes fifty-nine seconds. He had achieved a goal that nobody thought was possible. After Roger had broken the four-minute barrier, a strange thing happened. People began setting goals to run a mile in under four minutes and were succeeding, whereas previously they had tried and failed. In the three years after Roger Banister ran a mile in under four minutes, sixteen other runners had done the same thing. So my question to you is: what is your psychological barrier? What is your 'four-minute mile'? What is keeping you from breaking through it?

The point I am trying to get across is to be very careful to not let the limiting beliefs of others affect the goals you set, because what you can achieve is up to you and not up to others around you. What is stopping you from reaching your goals? If it is limiting beliefs, then you are talking yourself out of success. Now don't get confused: if you have a goal within the next two weeks to be a millionaire with no business up and running or no solid plan, then of course that is delusional – but in terms of the language we want to use, I would personally steer away from the word realistic as it only limits your way of thinking. The idea of realistic is something that has been imposed on each and every person by society, which then impacts your subjective way of viewing life – although to some extent 'realistic' does need to be considered, because a goal that is almost a fantasy can lead to demotivation and frustration if not achievable. What I am really trying to get across is that you should push yourself beyond your current realms of belief, as you can do more than you currently imagine.

If you want realistic results, you will do something realistic. If you want good results, you will do something that is good. If you want great results, you will do something great. If you want to totally dominate the industry you are in, then your way of thinking to the majority of people will be totally unrealistic. If you share these kinds of ideas with people and they have a differing viewpoint, then you are most likely on the right path.

'Impossible is just a big word thrown around by small men who find it easier to live in the world they've been given than to explore the power they have to change it. Impossible is not a fact. It's an opinion. Impossible is not a declaration. It's a dare. Impossible is potential. Impossible is temporary. Impossible is nothing.'

- Muhammad Ali

4. The 10 Steps to Goal Setting

The 10 Steps to Goal Setting is a formula I have refined over many years of goal setting. I have personally found that it focuses me and brings structure when achieving goals.

Each step will provide you with an organised plan of action to make sure that any given goal has been written out in a way that will allow you to reach your goals efficiently and effectively.

One of the reasons I have found this approach so effective is because of the positive language that is used in the present tense, making you feel as if you are already there.

The aim of this section of the book is to get you to be as effective as possible when goal setting. Without further ado, let's begin.

How to start

'All successful people are big dreamers. They imagine what their future could be, ideal in every respect, and then they work every day toward their distant vision, that goal or purpose.' Brian Tracy

Start off by imagining that there are no limitations on what you can be, have or do. Imagine that you have all the time and money, all the friends and contacts, all the education and experience that you need to accomplish any goal you set for yourself. Imagine that you could wave a magic wand and make your life perfect in each of the four key areas of life.

If your life was perfect in each area, what would it look like?

Income - how much do you want to earn this year, next year and five years from today?

Family - What kind of lifestyle do you want to create for yourself and your family?

Health - How would your health be different if you could have it the way you wanted it?

Net Worth - How much do you want to save and accumulate in your working life?

Exercise: Three Goal Method – in less than thirty seconds, write down your three most important goals in life. Do it right now.

1. _____

2. _____

3. _____

The reason behind this is because when you write it down without having time to think about it, what is written is more likely to be a true and accurate reflection of what you most desire.

'The way to get started is to quit talking and begin doing.'
- Walt Disney

5. Step 1: Set a Date

Deadlines

Deadlines are key when goal setting as without a timeframe, the unconscious brain is likely to lack the motivation to push you to meet your target on time. Have you ever been given a deadline at work? You work harder to meet the deadline as you don't want to run over. Your unconscious mind will do the self same thing when goal setting.

Imagine your unconscious mind is a little person on your shoulder, constantly reminding you to do something. He or she will continuously remind you to work on your goals and keep you on track without you even realising.

I myself have noticed this when goal setting. I set my '10 things I want to be, do and have' goals (which you will see later in this book) a year ago and forgot that I had written some of them down as there were so many and some were particularly small. When revisiting these goals months later, I realised I have achieved them without consciously putting effort into it. This is because my unconscious mind has kept me on track and pushed me to work towards a goal and make it happen without me being aware of it. The power of the unconscious brain is amazing when you review your goals and see how far you have come. If for some reason you don't achieve your goal by the deadline, simply set a new deadline. There are no unreasonable goals, only unreasonable deadlines.

Exercise Four: The Theory of Constraints – There is always one limiting factor or constraint that sets the speed at which you achieve your goal; what is it for you? For each of the three goals you have written above, write down a deadline by which you would like to achieve these goals and what the constraint is, whether it be seeing things through, being consistent, etc.

An example of this could be:
Goal - To become 10% body fat with lean muscle
Deadline - On or before 31.12.2017
Constraint - Temptation of fast food, cravings, procrastination

1. Deadline_____

    Constraint_____

2. Deadline_____

    Constraint_____

3. Deadline_____

    Constraint_____

The 80/20 Rule applies to constraints: 80% of the reasons that are holding you back from achieving your goals come from within yourself. They may be a lack of motivation, that you tend to be a procrastinator, a lack of skills, or not having the necessary knowledge required.

Only 20% of the reasons you are not achieving your goals are external to you. For example, one of the reasons that applies to the example I have given above is long days at work. This is usually your 'excuse factor' that you will give yourself to get out of working on your goals. I don't want you to rely on these excuses, and in the majority of cases you are able to overcome them. Obviously if you are working sixteen-hour days, then going to the gym may be difficult, but there is always time to prioritise the things that mean the most to you, aligning your priorities with your goals. In this case, those who work the nine to five may use the excuse that they have little time to go to the gym. However, a one-hour workout is only 4.16% of your day. When you put your 'excuse' into perspective, there is usually little reason to use it as an excuse.

This method can be used to counteract the majority of external constraints, as they are usually easy to overcome.

However, if for one day or one week you are required to work overtime which means you cannot get to the gym, don't allow yourself to become frustrated. This is not you not being able to achieve your goals; it is just an external factor that is a slight constraint. It's important to know it's okay if you're not 100% motivated every single day. There will be days that take you off-track, but you need to start each day fresh and rebalance yourself, so you will always be moving towards your goals.

Always start with yourself as it is the majority 80% constraint that appears to work against you.

This immediately demonstrates the importance of working on yourself as it is far more important to begin with how you can improve your chances before you start worrying about the 20% of external matters.

'A dream written down with a date becomes a goal'
- Greg S. Reid

6. Step 2: Detail is Key

Write it out in specific and precise detail

When setting goals it is important to write it out in as much detail as you possibly can as this focuses your mind on what you really want.

Example: a bad way of setting your goal
Goal: I want a Porsche by the end of next year. I want to save 10% of my wages every month to have a deposit for it.

Example: a good way of setting your goal
Goal: I own my Porsche 911 GT3 RS on or before 31st December 2018. It has 500 horse power at 8250 rpm and has a top speed of 193 mph. It does 0-60 in 3.1 seconds and its fuel consumption in the city is 14 mpg. The colour of my Porsche is Lava Orange, with black/lava orange leather interior and lava orange seat belts. It has comfortable full bucket seats and auto-dimming mirrors with integrated rain sensors. It has heated seats and air conditioning, with painted air vent slats to match the rest of the car. It has a Porsche doppelkupplung transmission which includes a 7-speed dual-clutch gearbox and a PDK SPORT button so I can drive in either automatic mode or using manual shift controls. My Porsche has 9.5J x 20inch GT3 RS platinum wheels on the front and 12.5J x 21inch GT3 RS platinum wheels on the back. Its base price is $175,900.

Can you see how different they are?

When you order a takeaway, you would not just ask for a pizza. You would ask for a mozzarella pizza, with a tomato and garlic base, chestnut mushrooms, green peppers and red onions, with a cheese-stuffed crust. The same goes for a car or for any given goal. You make it as specific as possible so that you work towards exactly what you want.

Here's a worksheet to help you focus when writing down your goals that combines the first two steps. It is important to sign your name on your goals so that you feel committed to it; like signing a contract, you are committing to your goals in the same way.

Date:_____

<u>Step 2: Detail is Key</u>

Goal_____

_____

_____

_____

_____

_____

_____

_____

_____

_____

Signature:_____

'I always wanted to be somebody, but now I realise I should have been more specific.'
- Lily Tomlin

7. Step 3: Manageable Steps

When setting goals it's important to have structure in how you set the goals themselves.

A great way to start is with small steps. If we have a goal that requires a big step, it can be daunting and can make us procrastinate regarding the tasks at hand. What we tend not to realise is that, by making just small steps each day/week and in this way breaking the process down, we can make serious progression towards our goals.

This step gets the ball rolling and helps you to see the light at the end of the tunnel – and that reaching it is possible. Let's have an example: let's say your goal is to own a Lamborghini.

Small steps for this big goal may be as follows:
• Call dealer to find the exact price of the car/deposit needed and what the monthly payments will be.
• Work out how you can offset the payments through offering a service of some kind e.g. if it's £2,000 a month for the car and you can do some affiliate marketing that makes you £2,000 a month, you are offsetting the car payments.
• Work out how much it will cost you per year.
• Work out how much it will cost you to run per month with fuel, insurance and road tax.

In this way you end up with a set figure and you know exactly how much money you need to either make or save.

You can now forecast from your current savings and earnings how long it will take, and can then set a date.

It is likely that to achieve this goal you're going to need to push yourself out of your comfort zone.

Daily small step: write down five goals to achieve that day that will push you closer towards the longer term goal e.g. 'I will close a deal to earn myself £500 commission'.

Weekly small step: spend two hours on affiliate marketing scheme to generate £2,000 per month to offset the monthly payments.
Monthly small step: transfer £1,000 a month of your current earnings into a separate account that is allocated for the deposit of £20,000 for the car.

You can now see how this slowly but surely pushes you towards achieving this goal, just by having a step-by-step plan. This may seem simple, yet millions of people don't do it. It's just as easy to do it as not to do it. Which is why only less than 10% of people continuously and habitually set goals and push themselves to achieve them.

Even within this 10%, not all will write down goals, which is why many of these people will not achieve the goals they set in the first place. They are those who are slightly more ambitious, with a clearer vision of where they want to go. But without a set plan, and without a hard copy of their goal, more often than not they will not achieve it.

There needs to be an equilibrium between breaking down the steps too far or not enough; as both have positives and negatives. Breaking down your goals into loads of small steps is good, because you have a clear idea of exactly how you will get there – but it can be demotivating if you break it down too much, as you may not meet every step exactly on time.

Larger and fewer steps can be more motivating as you have longer to achieve them, which can make them seem more attainable; however this can cause you to lose focus on exactly how to get there.

So a happy medium is needed: a good balance. How I found a good balance was to set daily goals but keep them small – something I will go over in the 'Daily Goals' chapter later in the book.

Goal: _____

_____

Manageable steps:

1 _____

_____

2 _____

_____

3 _____

_____

4 _____

_____

5 _____

_____

6 _____

_____

7 _____

_____

8 _____

_____

'Life is a series of steps. Things are done gradually. Once in a while there is a giant step. But most of the time we are taking small, insignificant steps on the stairway of life.'
- Ralph Ransom

8. Step 4: Identify Skills and Knowledge Required

One of the main pitfalls that people make when goal setting is that they get so focused on having or wanting a goal, they forget that in order to achieve it they may have to learn something or even become a different person.

You can't just get through life winging it and hoping for the best, as the goal will remain out of your reach.

The first thing to do is to identify who your mentors are. Who are the people you can look up to – maybe even speak to, if you are lucky enough – and who can bring you closer to achieving your goal? For example, if you want to be a successful businessman, one of your mentors/role models may be Richard Branson. To be like him, and to help you to become as successful as him, you would need to look at the skills he holds, that either you don't have or you need to work on to help project you towards your goals. A mentor could also be someone that you know: a college or university tutor, a successful member of your family, or maybe a friend.

Next, you would need to look at what specific skill(s) you require in order to achieve your goal. If you want to learn to play the guitar, a skill you require would be to read music. Although the ability to play the guitar is a skill itself, other skills can impact on the learning process, and a lack of these skills can hinder you on your path to reaching your goal.

You need to be specific when identifying the skills required. If you want to design your own brand, you can't just say 'I need to be more creative'. GET SPECIFIC! For this example you may want to consider a course in illustration to learn how to do that.

At this stage, you will also need to identify what knowledge is needed to be able to achieve your goal. For example, when starting a business you would need (at least to begin with) a basic business knowledge. Therefore the best way to start to acquire this knowledge, if you don't already have it, would be to buy and read a book on how to set up a business. This may seem simple but this is how great goals are achieved. First you need to ask yourself what simple, specific, basic skills and knowledge you require to get you there. One small step at a time.

Once the skills and knowledge have been identified, you need to write out in small steps how you will get there. If there is certain knowledge you need to obtain, is it freely available or do you need to get it from someone in particular? Therefore the first step to write down would be 'Meet Mr Bremner for a coffee meeting and discuss the marketing behind a new brand'. It is important to acknowledge whether specific knowledge is needed from a particular person to achieve your goal; therefore when writing out these steps you must be specific, even to the point of using that person's name. The reason behind this is because it gets you asking yourself more relevant questions about how you will get there. You will soon realise that it is in the questions that you ask yourself that you find great success.

Example: Shaun has already set a date, described his goal in detail and been specific with the goals that he wants to achieve. He has written out the manageable steps to set him on the path to starting his own business but he is now identifying the skills and knowledge required to get him there.

First he recognises that he has someone within his family – his uncle – whom he can look up to and see as a mentor, because the uncle is already successful in the line of business Shaun is getting into. Then he looks at the skills and knowledge difference between himself and his uncle to try to identify the information he will need to successfully enter this field. He should ask his uncle how he came about this knowledge and skill set and how Shaun too can do it.

Shaun would write this information out as a brainstorm separately until the information is ready to be written out using the steps.

Mentor – Uncle Chris

Knowledge – ask him questions:
1. *What are your top five books that you have read that moved you closer to the position of success you are in today?*
2. *Is there a specific book out of these five that was a game changer for you?*
3. *What supplier did you use in order to create your product, and can they facilitate my order?*

Skills – ask him questions:
1. *What are the top five skills you would say are most important in this industry?*
2. *Was it through experience that you developed them or are there any particular courses or exercises I can do to improve?*
3. *What is the most valuable skill you have that I can learn?*

Can you see what's happening here? Shaun is focusing on specific knowledge and skills he needs to do well in the industry he is entering. He is using his uncle to identify the skills and knowledge he himself doesn't hold in order to become a success. By using this process, he is cutting down the time that he could waste on researching the skills and knowledge needed, and gaining vital firsthand knowledge from someone who has made himself a success.

If his mentor was someone of whom it was not possible to ask these questions, Shaun would have to ask himself something like the below:

Mentor: Richard Branson

Knowledge:
1. What top five books has R. Branson publicly recommended as helping him on his path to success?
2. What one book has been publicised as his most highly recommended book?
3. What vital pieces of knowledge are within these books that I don't already have?

Skills:
1. What are the skills that R. Branson has for which he is most recognised in business?
2. In interviews he has done, has he suggested whether these skills were gained through experience or has he recommended particular ways to improve on these skills?
3. What does he consider to be his most valuable skill?

Now that Shaun has the answers to these questions, he will write them down with his goal as follows:

Knowledge and Skills

I am reading 'The Chimp Paradox' by Dr Steve Peters in order to gain the knowledge required to control my emotions within difficult business situations. This is going to ensure that I build good customer and supplier relations and move closer towards my goal of becoming successful in this field. I look up to both my uncle and Dr S Peters as mentors, as they both hold this knowledge.

I have enrolled in a course on illustration that I go to once a week as it fits comfortably around work. This is going to help me to build the skill required to design my products, which will move me closer towards my goal of being a fulltime business owner.

I have given one example each of skills and knowledge that Shaun could detail whilst writing out his goals. I must stress that there will not only be one skill and one section of knowledge needed to achieve your goals, and I urge you to be as specific and in-depth as possible within this section.

As you can see, not only does this section help you start acknowledging the skills and knowledge required, it prompts you to take action.

Possible Mentors:

1. _____   2. _____

3. _____   4. _____

Knowledge questions to ask:

1. _____

_____

2. _____

_____

3. _____

_____

Skills questions to ask:

1. _____

_____

2. _____

_____

3. _____

_____

Knowledge and Skills:

1. _____

_____

_____

2. _____

_____

_____

3. _____

_____

_____

4. _____

_____

_____

5. _____

_____

_____

6. _____

_____

_____

7. _____

_____

_____

8. _____

_____

_____

9. _____

_____

_____

10. _____

_____

_____

'Know, first,
who you are,
and then
adorn
yourself
accordingly.'
- Epictetus

9. Step 5: Identify Your Obstacles

This is one of my favourite sections. The majority of the time what you perceive to be obstacles are in fact not obstacles at all. The obstacles that may spring to mind when you first think of them are things like time, money, contacts, etc. However, the only real obstacle is yourself. Only when you realise that it is only you getting in the way of your goals and dreams can you begin to make what you want happen.

Taking responsibility is key because when you accept that it's you and only you holding yourself back, your mind begins to dig deep into your subconscious to adjust old patterns of thought and create new ones. Accepting responsibility triggers you to start asking empowering questions. When you develop this type of attitude you will always find your way around an obstacle. No matter what it is, that inner voice of yours will condition itself to think of another way round it. If you get stuck, do you just give up? Or do you pivot and accept it for what it is and move on? This is easier said than done, and granted, it took me a while to get good at this. Pivoting is a skill, as it is so very easy to get caught up in your business idea, for example, that you limit yourself by thinking your initial route is the only one. Be open-minded enough if you hit a road block to take a different route.

I like to consider the other things that stand in the way of you achieving your goals as 'minor hurdles'. Instead of viewing them as an 'obstacle' that is blocking your way, view them as a hurdle; the word in itself makes the task seem easier to overcome, as we leap forward.

Now let's start with examples of identifying hurdles. Here are three examples:

- **Parents** – Instinctively, most parents will want to protect their children so don't take it personally if they are not 100% supportive of your ideas at first... Example: Shaun is young and ambitious with a hunger for business. His parents care about him, so naturally want him to strive for a higher education and get good grades. Although they see his business plan as a good idea, they do not want him to leave school at sixteen to pursue a business instead of going to college and then onto university. Now this isn't one of the moments that you start thinking of your parents as a true obstacle and start resenting them; see them rather as a minor hurdle, because they want the best for you. If your parents are not that supportive of you being an entrepreneur then I'm not surprised as it's seen as 'risky'. Keeping your goals to yourself can sometimes be a good thing as nine out of ten times, once you have a solid plan and your parents see how serious you are, they will then support you.

- **Friends** – This again may seem a strange one but your friends can appear to be a hurdle on your way towards your goals. They can potentially hold you back. Accept this, don't question it, and move on. If they do not support you it will often be a reflection of their own insecurities rather than your own... Example: Shaun is very fitness- and health-orientated. He likes to work out and eat healthily in order to maintain his body and keep it in a good condition. However, Shaun's friends do not share this interest. They enjoy eating at fast food restaurants before going out on a Saturday night to drink. This is often Shaun's only chance to see his friends due to separate work and other commitments. Therefore Shaun may often go along on these nights with his friends, which will impact on his fitness goal as his friends have no interest in many social activities that he enjoys.

- **Capital** – This may seem like a difficult hurdle to overcome because, with money, it's either there or it isn't. However, if you think of it like this, you will find it difficult to overcome it. This brings me onto empowering questions that will help you to overcome hurdles such as this.

46

Empowering Questions

Generally as humans we focus on the negative. I am sure we've all fallen into that trap, which reminds me of the old saying 'when it rains, it pours'. What about changing that thought process by managing your 'inner narrator'? What if when it rains, it just rains? This comes in the form of acceptance, which is something you're going to want to hold as a value; when accepting that goals may take time, you can still be incredibly successful at reaching them.

A change of language can make all the difference. Make a conscious effort to understand how you speak to yourself and ask yourself questions that are going to empower you, to bring you closer to your goals, rather than further away. I honestly believe that in each of us is a hidden genius; sometimes we just need a kick up the backside to unlock it. Asking yourself empowering questions not only helps you to think positively, but it gets you asking the right questions, and in turn finding the desired answer.

Ask something one way, and you'll end up with limiting beliefs, thoughts that resemble the stereotypical 'I'm never going to be able to buy that'. Ask another way and you'll find yourself having thoughts like 'What books are successful people reading right now on how to achieve multiple sources of income?' This is how you tap into new thought patterns. My idea and rationale behind this is that, deep down, we already know what we need to do – we just have to start asking the right questions. I want you all to remember: '*it only costs zero pounds to think like a millionaire.*'

Asking empowering questions is key, as it focuses your mind on thinking about the means of reaching your goal. It gets you asking the right questions, thus pushing you towards your goals much faster.

Instead of asking 'how will I afford to buy that Ferrari?' you need to ask yourself 'how can I triple my income in order to be able to buy my Ferrari?'

Instead of asking 'how will I ever do that?' ask yourself 'what skill(s) do I want to become really good at? What can I do today to start to master them?'

Let's say you want to learn to play the guitar. The best way to ask yourself how would be to structure it in this way: 'What video on YouTube can I watch today in order to start learning to play the guitar? Where can I find a good guitar teacher?'

You are your only obstacle

Here are the most common seven ways that can lead to self-sabotage:

1. **Trying to do too much** – Although in the beginning writing a long list of goals may make you feel motivated and driven and seem impressive, this could in fact hinder your ability to achieve them. Your mind will become so muddled and will be so stretched between them all that you will not have enough time to focus on each of them for long enough to make sufficiently big steps towards reaching them. This will lead to you becoming demotivated, and to feeling overwhelmed and frustrated, and you may begin to procrastinate. Have you ever been in a situation where you have so much to do that you end up doing nothing at all? This isn't to say you can't be driven and set lots of goals, but there needs to be a balance.

2. **Remaining in your comfort zone** – It is human nature to remain in a position where you feel comfortable and safe. Have you ever stayed in a job for longer than you know you should just because you knew what to expect and what was coming? When you moved out from your parents' house(s), did it take you longer than you had initially planned, and did you do it later in life than you had originally thought you would? This is because when we are in a known environment it feels safer, and therefore we find it difficult to stretch the boundaries and break the mould because we become complacent.

3. **Being stuck in the past** – If you continue to dwell on the past – on what you could have done differently and/or better – you may miss the opportunity to make the change today to live a better tomorrow. If you allow the past to consume you, then today will eventually become tomorrow/next week/next month/next year, and you will waste your life on 'shoulda, coulda, woulda's'. It's important to be aware of this so not to continue as a broken record.

4. **Not taking consistent action and procrastinating** – Have you ever said to yourself 'oh, I have ages to do that, I can do it tomorrow'? Procrastination and inconsistently taking action towards your goals is a major hindrance to reaching them. You can find yourself forever living on 'Tomorrow Island', where everything is always pushed back a day but in reality never gets done. By setting daily goals, which you will read about more in a later chapter in this book, you can keep your mind focused and be continually working on your goals on a daily basis.

5. **Fear** – The fear of the unknown and the fear of taking risks can stop you working towards your goals altogether. It makes you feel uncomfortable so in order to overcome it, you need to discover the source of the fear itself. What is it that you are really afraid of? Fear can convince you to stay where you are in case you fail and can cripple you when attempting to achieve your goals. Fear is just False Evidence Appearing Real. You have two options: Let fear force you into walking away from your goals, or take a bold stand against fear and let it serve you, fuel you, and push you on.

6. **Pessimistic voices** – The analogy of the devil and angel on your shoulders comes to mind. The devil will attempt to poison your mind and will show you all the reasons why you cannot reach your goal. As humans we are psychologically programmed to remember bad events/feelings/emotions that we have experienced. Therefore we are instinctively more likely to remember all the reasons against doing something rather than the reasons to do it, which may in fact outweigh all the negatives.

7. **You don't give a f***** – This is when you have set yourself a goal, maybe to impress others or because it is something that you think you should want, but that in reality you do not want at all. You think it sounds good and you like the idea of it but in reality, if it was not to come about, you wouldn't care. If you find yourself telling yourself 'I just need to get motivated' then it's not as important to you as you may have first thought. This could quite simply be down to the fact that you don't hold the values required in order to get that goal, or you don't care enough. Quite simply, you just don't give a f***.

These are seven dreadful ingredients that lead to a cocktail of disaster, leaving a very sour taste in your mouth. If you're sitting there thinking that this is you and you are unsure what to do, this is easily and simply combatted, and I'll show you how. Daily goals, values and affirmations (discussed later in this book) will help you to tackle this cocktail of negativity and will lead you to overcoming your main obstacle – yourself. As well as the daily goals method, when writing out your obstacles and hurdles in full you should positively word the solutions.

Example: Shaun has issues speaking to his parents about his goals and ambitions. This is because they feel that the best thing for him would be to continue within education as far as possible rather than leaving school at sixteen to start a business, thus taking a big risk. It is important for him to notice that his parents are only doing this because they care, even though their wish may not be the best thing for him. Therefore he recognises this as a hurdle on the path to achieving his goal.

He WOULD NOT write: '*My parents are a hurdle as I cannot discuss my dreams with them*', as this brings negativity into his goal setting, which could have a detrimental effect.

He WOULD write: '*I am focusing on discussing my ideas with likeminded individuals who can give me subjective and unbiased feedback that will continue to push me towards my goals*'.

Ultimately, after seeing what we have discussed above it is more visible that the things that appear to stand in your way are minor hurdles, and in reality the only obstacle to achieving your goal is you and the story you tell yourself on a daily basis about why you can't do something.

Exercise: Identify the biggest five hurdles standing in your way of achieving your goal, and address them with a solution.

1. Hurdle_____

    Solution_____

2. Hurdle_____

    Solution_____

3. Hurdle_____

    Solution_____

4. Hurdle_____

    Solution_____

5. Hurdle_____

    Solution_____

'When obstacles arise, you change your direction to reach your goal; you do not change your decision to get there.'
- Zig Ziglar

10. Step 6: People to Associate With

If you read this section and start getting angry, I ask you to read the whole chapter as there is a lot to take from it. It is very easy for me to push people's buttons within this section and to touch on nerves, as a lot of what I'm about to say is not what many people want to hear. But it is what they need to hear. If you do not get the wrong people out of your life you'll never meet the right ones.

In this section I take you through the importance of surrounding yourself with likeminded people who have either had the same success as you, or have had the success that you desire and wish to learn from. One of the biggest mistakes we make is that we fail to realise is how important our social circle is and the effect it has on our goals. I have seen and experienced firsthand the effects of 'friends' subtly bringing you down to their level. The harsh truth is that the majority of friends and sometimes even family are not going to be happy for your success. The more quickly you accept that, the more quickly you can get on with the show and start focusing on bringing your goals closer.

Have you ever met a group of people and thought that they all seem to be almost clones of each other? They have similar nicknames, speak in similar slang and think the same, while holding very similar views on life. This may start to sound familiar. What happens now if you are a member of that group but start to develop different thought patterns? You become more curious about goals, building businesses and income creation. It is very likely that when you share your views, your friends will impose their common views and beliefs on what they think you can and can't achieve. This is because they see you as similar to themselves and cannot see themselves reaching these goals. Now here is the crazy part... you listen to them. This is the very thing that is sucking away at your ambition.

Think about it... if you were to hang around with Richard Branson every day for a week, how do think you'd feel about what is possible in life? You'd be embarrassed to say 'I think this can't be done' etc. Why? Because you know he would laugh, as he thinks in a way that makes almost everything possible. Now we do not all have the luxury of being around such great minds like Richard Branson but we do have choices about who we associate with. A choice about who we spend our time and energy on. Unfortunately your friends will not be paying your bills in the future so make sure you're not having your mind poisoned by someone else's limiting beliefs.

Who you spend your time with will have a great impact in your life. If you're hanging around with people who are on a downwards spiral in life, have no ambition, no drive, and no interest in changing, they are likely to be dragging you down with them. 'Walk with the wise and become wise, for a companion of fools suffers harm.' – Proverbs 13:20. Whatever quality, good or bad, it will rub off on you.

On a lighter note, let us focus on the benefits of being around likeminded, positive people.

- Encouragement
- They push you towards your goals
- They are authentically happy for you
- They keep you on track and pick you up when you're feeling down or stressed
- They give you honest advice rather than what you want to hear
- They will support your projects

The list could go on but the key thing to take away from this is that you can spend ten years going round in circles, hanging around with

Leeches, or you can surround yourself with secure likeminded people who will push you ever closer to your goals and support you.

Here's the good news. If you hang around generous people, you'll become more generous. If you hang around with successful people, you'll become successful. The same good qualities will start to rub off on you and will become a part of your life. That's why it is so important to be selective about whom you spend your time with.

Red and Green Flags

We need to consider the 'red flags' of the people we associate with and how these should deter us. We shouldn't hang around with people who are horrible to their spouses, family, kids, friends, etc; we have to set these boundaries. This is because if we associate with these people they may begin to infect us without us being aware of it, and even without their own intent. Have you ever sat and listened to someone speak about something, feeling perfectly happy beforehand but after listening to their story you hold anger and resentment against the particular person or topic that has been discussed? Even though, in reality, it has no impact on you at all? It will work in the same way. For example, your co-worker appears to be unhappy in their relationship and so they vent to you. This starts making you think more about your own relationships; things that seemed small begin to seem larger, and you begin to vent. You leave the conversation angry and feeling down about your own relationship when in reality there is nothing wrong with it. Surrounding yourself with negative people and the wrong type of people will do this to you in a bigger and more impactful way.

Now that we have red flags covered, let's move onto the green flags. These are the characteristics you see in people whom you definitely want in your life. The people who possess these infections characteristics generally have a particular type of demeanour. You will feel positive vibes from them the moment you meet them. Naturally, this often brings out the best in you, drawing out your own good qualities. A green flag characteristic could be self-assurance.

Surrounding yourself with someone who is self-assured will lead to you becoming more confident and positive in your own thoughts and ideas, just as they are. Being around someone like that will make you question why you are not like this person; it will start a process within your mind of seeking out the similarities and differences between you and that person, which will drive you to become more like them. It is important to not be a copycat of someone else but rather to recognise characteristics you do not yet have that will help you on your journey. Life is too short to waste your valuable time with the wrong people. This is one of the main reasons I see that gets people off course. The more successful you become, the more selective you have to be and the closer your circle will become.

The hardest thing you'll have to do is letting go of people who shouldn't be in your life. It doesn't mean they are bad people; it's just they are not on the same journey as you. Sometimes you have to love people from a distance. I am not saying you should cut off your family members and all your friends, but sometime you need to be mindful of how many hours you are spending with a certain person. Reanalyse the amount of time you spend with the negative 'red flag' people in your life, as they will not push you on your way to reaching your goals.

Ask yourself these questions: 'How many times have I spent time with people that I know (and knew at the time) aren't good for me? Did I only spend time with them because I didn't want to hurt their feelings? Have I ever been in a situation where I have made plans with someone but didn't really want to go, without knowing a real reason, and therefore made an excuse and put it off?' The answer to this final question may be very clear. It may be your intuition telling you that this person is not good for you and that they are not helping you on your way to achieving your goal(s) in life.

Be a giver (to a certain extent)

It is good to be a giver. It is good to be generous. However, a giver who gives too much can be left with empty pockets.

Let's say that your friend needs your help. He is demotivated, lacks ambition, is feeling down and seems to be spiralling into a black hole. You, being you, want to help as much as you can. You give him advice as to the best books to read to boost his mood, give him advice on audio books, speakers, YouTube clips to watch and listen to. You give him advice on how to better his life in his job and his relationship, and he goes away seeming motivated and inspired. A week later you check in on him and he is back to square one; he feels the same as how he felt before he spoke to you initially and has followed none of your advice. Therefore you, again being you, give him further advice. And the pattern repeats, again and again. But what happens in the end?

You have given him every bit of advice you can think of. And instead of walking away as the positive, motivated individual you are, you feel drained and negative and as if you have let him down. You feel guilt when in reality this person has not followed one piece of advice you have given them. RED FLAG. This is not the sort of person you want in your life. They may be your friend, and you may want to help them as much as you can, but they will drain the positivity out of you.

Think of it like this. You have a circle. It is filled with positivity. When you work on your own projects you take positivity from the circle and push it into the work you are doing. You reap the rewards, whether it be money or gratitude, and positivity is put back into the circle.

However, whilst helping your friend, you are taking this positivity from your circle and pushing it into him. He is then doing nothing with it, which means there is no positivity to put back into your circle. Your circle becomes smaller and more deflated and in the end there is no positivity left for you.

Remember this: you are not responsible for other people's happiness, you are only responsible for your own. It is imperative that you associate with your green flags.

Exercise: Red and Green Flags

This exercise may seem a bit brutal, but there is a reason behind it. Take the five people whom you spend the most time with. Analyse their red flag characteristics and their green flag characteristics. Is it skewed on one side, particularly for any of these people? Those who are skewed mostly to the green flag side are those with whom you should be spending most of your time. These are the driven people who will help push you towards your goals.

This is – and I'm not going to lie to you – going to be a horrible process. Analysing your best friends can be heartbreaking if you realise that in reality they are not the best people to associate with. And this is why I must stress again: I AM NOT ASKING YOU TO CUT OFF YOUR FRIENDS COMPLETELY. I'm just asking you to reanalyse the amount of time you spend with people depending on to what extent they will help you to achieve your goals.

Examples:

Red Flags: cynical, lazy, unambitious, uninspired, dishonest, selfish, closed-minded, unreliable, ignorant, immoral, jealous, pessimistic, etc.

Green Flags: ambitious, inspired, honest, giving, open-minded, reliable, moral, optimistic, empowering, committed, self-aware, courageous.

Below is a worksheet that can be printed five times to complete this exercise if you wish to do it on paper, or it can be done in your own personal journal.

Person _____

Red Flags: Green Flags:

_____   _____

_____   _____

_____   _____

_____   _____

_____   _____

_____   _____

_____   _____

_____   _____

_____   _____

_____   _____

_____   _____

_____   _____

_____   _____

_____   _____

_____   _____

'Beware of the company you keep. See that you associate with the right type of people.'
- Dada Vaswani

11. Step 7: What Is in it for You and Why?

In this section it is very important to clearly identify what is in it for you and why. Let me explain...

When you know your 'why' – when you know deep down the reason for the goal – you will push through the hurdles and the roadblocks and much more.

The main benefit I have found from this process is that it gives me clarity as to why I am trying to reach this goal, and this gives me the extra momentum I need to get there. Just wanting something isn't a good enough reason to be trying to get there; a completely clear and specific reason in your mind will enable you to overcome most obstacles on your path. Sometimes you may even find that the goal isn't as important to you as you first thought, which saves you a lot of time chasing a goal that you, in fact, do not really want.

Exercise: 10 reasons why

I use this exercise myself to help me differentiate between goals I really want to achieve and fabricated goals that I only think I want to meet.

Write out ten reasons why you want to achieve this goal, and ten things that are 'in it for you' when you get there. The first few will be easy, but as you go along you might find that you have to spend longer than you expected on completing this task.

Why do I want to achieve this goal?

1. _____

_____

2. _____

_____

3. _____

_____

4. _____

_____

What is in it for me?

1. _____

_____

2. _____

_____

3. _____

_____

4. _____

_____

Do you want a Lamborghini? If you were presented with £300,000 today, would you go to the dealer right away or would you stop and think 'what do I actually want?' The majority of people want to show everyone what their goals are to impress people they don't like. Not every person wants a supercar or a Rolex or a penthouse in central London. Others have goals such as being free from the nine to five, having more time to spend with their kids or more time to play golf with friends, or just wanting to build businesses. Your values are perfect for you and there is really no need to set goals to impress others. The most refreshing thing you can feel is filtering out what goals are truly important to you because this can be the most relieving feeling. You'll feel a sense of clarity and have extra motivation to succeed. You need to know the end reason of what is really in it for you, and once you have that you'll do great things, pushing through any hurdle that comes your way.

Example: Shaun used to find it difficult to achieve his goals. He felt the goals he was focusing on were to impress others, which left him lacking the needed motivation to propel himself towards them. After being frustrated that he was not getting where he needed to, there came a moment of enlightenment. He sat down in a quiet place and started to think and have honest conversations with himself. He came to a realisation that he was doing it for the wrong reasons.

Initially, he had thought what he wanted was to own a sports car: an Audi R8, to be specific. But when he sat down and really thought about it, he realised this was not aligned with his core values: it was a goal he had put upon himself due to the feeling of needing to impress others. He came to the realisation that what he was more interested in was reinvesting the capital he had already earned into further building his business, and any remaining cash he would prefer to spend on living a healthy and active lifestyle. He was much more easily able to answer the questions 'why do I want to achieve this goal' and 'what's in it for me' when he was able to specifically identify goals that meant more to him.

I cannot stress highly enough how much you need to have clarity with your 'whys'. They need to be at the forefront of your mind. Your whys need to be bigger than the hurdles you may face, otherwise you will not overcome them. If you have ever felt like this, frustrated in the past with your goals, and may have even felt stuck as to why you're not pushing through, the majority of the time it's because you haven't figured out why you truly want the goal in the first place. By doing this exercise you'll save yourself a lot of time and will finally feel that clarity that you're striving towards what you truly want. I encourage you to do this exercise for each goal to ensure it is what you really want.

'When you have clarity of intention, the universe conspires with you to make it happen.'
- Fabienne Fredrickson

12. Step 8: What Are You Prepared to Give Up?

Identifying what you are prepared to give up is key within the goal-setting and goal-achieving process. This is where many people fall down, as they are unprepared to sacrifice in order to achieve the goal they have set. If you are saving for the deposit of your first home or any other goal, it is likely you will have to sacrifice going out with your friends, cinema trips and eating out with your partner, and new clothes and other expenditure on yourself. For some, this sacrifice of enjoyment and treating oneself is too much, which is why they do not achieve their goal of owning their own home, or why it takes them far longer to raise the capital for the deposit than they initially planned. It's not just sacrificing money and spending money; it's also about time. There are only twenty-four hours in the day, seven days in the week, and fifty-two weeks in the year. You will need to be prepared to reduce the amount of time you spend doing other things in order to achieve your goals.

> Example: Shaun works fulltime. He works a nine to five job, five days a week, and it takes him approximately an hour to travel to work and home each way so he is out of the house for ten hours of the day. He then sleeps for seven hours a night. That is already seventeen hours of the day and ninety-nine hours of a 168-hour week gone. Shaun likes to go to the gym so he spends one and a half hours five times a week exercising. There are now only sixty-one and a half hours of the week remaining. He spends two hours every day showering and preparing his food and eating. Now there are forty-seven and a half hours left. He spends six hours on a night out with his friends, seven hours (one hour a day) playing on his PS4, fourteen hours (two hours a day) watching TV with his partner, five hours on an evening out with his partner for dinner and to the cinema, six hours on a Saturday and Sunday spending

time with his family, going for lunch with his partner, going to the beach/shopping/etc, and finally half an hour every day practising his guitar. This is his time up.

Shaun wants to set up a side business in order to raise capital to buy himself and his partner their first home. He has recognised that he needs to be more efficient with his time as he will need to dedicate time to setting up and growing his business. He has consciously made the decision to reduce his TV time by one hour per day, to reduce the time he spends on the PS4 weekly to just two hours on the weekend, and to sacrifice a night out with his friends three times a month, now only going to one every four weeks. He has dedicated two hours every Saturday and Sunday in the morning to working on his business, as four hours each of the two days is still quite a lot of time to go and see his family and go out with his partner for the afternoon, and to only go out with his partner for dinners and to the cinema every other week. Instead they will spend three hours getting a takeaway and watching a film.

On the weeks he is not out with his partner or his friends, he has freed up:

TV time -	7 hours
PS4 time -	5 hours
Night out -	6 hours
Weekend -	4 hours
Night in -	2 hours
Total -	24 hours

He has now freed up the equivalent of a day per week that he can focus on his side business.

On the weeks he is out with his partner, but not out with his friends, he has freed up:

TV time	7 hours
PS4 time -	5 hours
Night out -	6 hours
Weekend -	4 hours
Total -	22 hours

On the weeks he is not out with his partner, but out with his friends, he has freed up:

TV time -   7 hours
PS4 time -   5 hours
Weekend -   4 hours
Night in -   2 hours
Total -   18 hours

On the weeks he is out with his partner and out with his friends, he has freed up:

TV time -   7 hours
PS4 time -   5 hours
Weekend -   4 hours
Total -   16 hours

Even in his worst case scenario week, where he is spending eleven hours out with his friends and his partner, he is still able to free up sixteen hours in the week to work on his business.

It's very likely that one of the main reasons you're not achieving your goals is the excuses you're telling yourself. Have you ever said to yourself 'oh, I just don't have the time'? Well, the example above shows that most of you WILL have the time. Efficiently managing your time can free up more spare time than you think; it's just a matter of making the sacrifices required in order to do so.

Exercise: Cutting your time.

Below is an exercise that divides life into its main sections. Fill in the sections with how much time you spend per week on each activity and you'll soon see how much free time you really have.

How I spend my time now (fill in blanks with other time-consuming activities):

	M	T	W	T	F	S	S	Total
Work								
Travel								
Eating								
Sleeping								
Showering and getting ready								
Out with friends								
Out with partner								
Family time								
TV								

How I want to/will now spend my time (fill in blanks with other time-consuming activities):

	M	T	W	T	F	S	S	Total
Work								
Travel								
Eating								
Sleeping								
Showering and getting ready								
Out with friends								
Out with partner								
Family time								
TV								

I understand that sacrifice is hard, but if you're not willing to cut back on the non-necessities then it's going to make achieving your goals more difficult, particularly if they are time-consuming.

Sacrifice is absolutely necessary if you want to get where you want to be in life. Whether that be financially, physically, spiritually or in any other way, sacrifice is key. Any role model you have ever looked up to will have had to sacrifice time, pleasure and many other things at some point or many points in their life to get where they are. If you want to follow in their footsteps and achieve success in all areas of your life, then you need something that is going to give you your edge. Many people overcomplicate it, but the simple practical step above will help you to see what you really spend your time on. Many of you will be surprised at how much time you spend doing nothing. You may even be struggling to fill in the full twenty-four hours of the day as you're sometimes unaware of how you are really spending your time.

Imagine if you could give yourself a day – a full day a week – as Shaun did, to work towards your goal. Picture how quickly it would become a reality. A whole twenty-four hours a week, for fifty-two weeks of the year, is a massive 1,248 hours a year to work towards your goal. Now tell me you 'don't have the time'. Ask yourself 'how many goals are achievable within those hours?'

Offset your time

One good way to save time would be to multitask. If you don't want to give up either going to the gym or reading/listening to books, a good idea would be to combine them. Whilst in the gym, whether you are doing weights or on the treadmill, it would be time-efficient to listen to your audio book at the same time. (This would also work for housework.) Do you drive or use public transport to get to work? Would it be more time-efficient for you to get the train so you can reply to emails in the time that you would usually be driving? The key point here is that offsetting your time can make your day much more productive.

'If you don't sacrifice for what you want, what you want will be the sacrifice.'
- Unknown

13. Step 9: Affirmations

This is a small yet very effective step in the process of setting and achieving your goals. In the earlier section on psychology you saw what affirmations are and how the vocabulary used can be very influential on the effectiveness of this process. However, when setting goals it is highly important to ensure your stated affirmations closely linked to your goals. Although affirmations such as 'I attract an abundance of health, wealth and happiness' can be very effective in general life, if you have the specific goal of becoming 10% body fat, it is only loosely linked to the subject.

> Example: Shaun is very fitness-orientated. He has the goal of becoming 10% body fat and then to maintain a lean and toned physique. The most effective way to affirm this would be to write it down in this manner:
>
> I am 10% body fat on or before 1 December 2017.
> I am 10% body fat on or before 1 December 2017.
> I am 10% body fat on or before 1 December 2017.
> I am 10% body fat on or before 1 December 2017.
> I am 10% body fat on or before 1 December 2017.
> I am 10% body fat on or before 1 December 2017.
> I am 10% body fat on or before 1 December 2017.
> I am 10% body fat on or before 1 December 2017.
> I am 10% body fat on or before 1 December 2017.
> I am 10% body fat on or before 1 December 2017.
>
> I do HIIT training every day for 20 minutes.
> I do HIIT training every day for 20 minutes.
> I do HIIT training every day for 20 minutes.
> I do HIIT training every day for 20 minutes.
> I do HIIT training every day for 20 minutes.
> I do HIIT training every day for 20 minutes.

I do HIIT training every day for 20 minutes.
I do HIIT training every day for 20 minutes.
I do HIIT training every day for 20 minutes.
I do HIIT training every day for 20 minutes.

I am strong, lean, toned and feel in great shape.
I am strong, lean, toned and feel in great shape.
I am strong, lean, toned and feel in great shape.
I am strong, lean, toned and feel in great shape.
I am strong, lean, toned and feel in great shape.
I am strong, lean, toned and feel in great shape.
I am strong, lean, toned and feel in great shape.
I am strong, lean, toned and feel in great shape.
I am strong, lean, toned and feel in great shape.
I am strong, lean, toned and feel in great shape.

As already mentioned in the psychology section, writing out the affirmations ten times each solidifies them in your mind, thus focusing you further on your goal, and giving you a higher likelihood of you staying on track and therefore achieving your goals. This step comes at the very end of the fully written-out goal. After all of the previous eight steps have been completed fully, this is an added bonus to ensure you're moving in the right direction and doing everything within your power to achieve your goal.

You don't need to use the affirmations I've provided, you can make up your own, but you need to ensure they are positively written in the way explained in the psychology section of this book; this is key.

Seven-Day Affirmation Challenge

This is a really easy way to get you going, especially if you've never done affirmations before, and it's a fast way to create a habit. Commit yourself to writing down a minimum of five affirmations, five times, every single day. This will soon become a part of your routine and you'll quickly begin to see a difference in how you think and feel.

Exercise: Take one of your goals, and think of two specific and relevant affirmations that apply. Write them out in the correct format and language, keeping them positive and present.

Goal:

_____

_____

Affirmation 1:

1._____

_____

2._____

_____

3._____

_____

4._____

_____

5._____

_____

6._____

_____

7._____

_____

8._____

_____

9._____

_____

10._____

_____

Affirmation 2:

1._____

_____

2._____

_____

3._____

_____

4._____

_____

5._____

_____

6._____

7._____

8._____

9._____

10._____

'Affirmation without discipline is the beginning of delusion.'
- Jim Rohn

14. Step 10: Visualisation

Visualisation is the process of engaging your senses in order to make the goal feel closer and more real. I like to think of it as a type of meditation, where you are focusing your mind completely on your goal and visualising that the goal has already been achieved. It is a key component to get in touch with your goal on a more intimate level. I have personally used visualisation whilst setting the goal of writing this book. I imagined and pictured this book before I began writing it, and today here you are reading it.

Visualisation can be used to programme your mind and body into getting positive results. It has been said that visualisation and the mind hold an important role in the creation of experiences, and therefore the positive experiences created through visualisation can be the driving force to achieving your goals.

It is a form of rehearsal of your goal, mentally imagining the goal multiple times and rehearsing the feeling in your mind. Certain studies, such as *Emotional Memory Management: Positive Control Over Your Memory* by Joseph M. Carver, Ph.D., have shown that the brain doesn't know the difference between imagining something and actually doing it. In his work, Carver found that basketball players who practised shots for one month improved their skill by 24%, those who only mentally imagined practising their shots improved by 23%, and those who did nothing did not improve. The power of the mind truly is great when you can practise a skill mentally, without even touching a basketball, and improve almost as much as a group of people who have been practising for a month.

Now imagine your goal. Whether it be to be able to make twenty basketball shots in a row, be 10% body fat, own a Ferrari, or be a great business person, really truly imagine it. Picture it in your mind and your body will instinctively begin to work towards this target without your conscious control. You'll find yourself working harder in the gym, or feeling more motivated to finish business plans and set up meetings with potential investors, because your body and mind will already know what it feels like to be in that shape or to be that successful.

The five-minute rule

The most basic way of visualisation would be through five minutes of meditation. For five minutes every evening before you go to bed, ensure that you have some time to yourself. Begin to visualise yourself as the person who has already achieved that goal. Imagine looking at yourself in the mirror as an athletic individual, or picture looking down at yourself in a sharp suit on the way to your international business meeting. Whatever your goal is, visualise it.

Then again, for the first five minutes after you wake, repeat this process. Visualise exactly how your life will be when you have achieved this goal and visualise the happiness you will feel when you get there. This will be the strongest push you need towards your goals.

Get your senses involved

Visualising can sometimes be difficult if you have not experienced the particular sensation before. The best thing to do to overcome this difficulty is to get your senses involved.

Example: Shaun has always dreamed of owning a Porsche GT3. As he has never sat in one or driven one he is finding it difficult to visualise what it would be like to own one.

Therefore, he firstly uses YouTube to listen to the sound that a Porsche GT3 makes, then closes his eyes whilst sitting in his own car and listens to the sound of the rev of the engine, picturing that a Porsche GT3 is what he is sitting in.

> He then imagines the smell of the Porsche GT3. Does it have a new car small? Does it smell like a particular air freshener? He goes out to buy that air freshener and puts it in his own car.
>
> Next, he visits the Porsche garage to sit in and see and feel the car for himself.
>
> With all this newfound knowledge of the car it is easier for Shaun to use his five minutes and accurately visualise owning the car for himself.

With the information from the 'Detail is Key' chapter, visualisation can be a very simple but effective technique in bringing your goal closer to you. You have already stated specifically what your goal is, with great detail in every aspect of it; now use this information to picture it in your mind.

While you are reading this, take part in a small task for me.
Raise your hand.
Now raise it higher.
And now higher again.
And now even higher.

Why did you not raise it that high in the first place? When I first asked you to raise your hand, why did you not raise it as high as possible?

It's almost as if your initial thought of where you believe yourself to be is lower. Why were you not comfortable enough the first time to raise your hand as high as you could? Visualisation helps to continually push through the barrier of your belief system, helping you to imagine life in a greater way then you could before, breaking through that self-imposed threshold.

Exercise: Meditation and visualisation

Although five minutes of meditation can be somewhat effective towards achieving your goals, the more you are able to visualise the better.

Take your five senses: sight, touch, taste, sound and smell. Pick four of them (I understand that taste can be difficult to apply to many goals) and choose four ways that you will engage your senses to be able to better visualise your goal.

Example for Shaun and his car:
- Sight - go to a showroom and see the car. Look through the catalogues and select colours that I would want, specific features and add-ons that I would want on my car.
- Touch - sit in the car in the showroom and feel the steering wheel, gearstick, hand brake; press the pedals and be as hands-on as possible whilst sitting in the car.
- Sound - listen to the sound on Youtube, or take the car for a test drive or be driven around by the dealer.
- Smell - smell the new car smell or the smell of the air freshener; then go out and buy the air freshener and put it in my car.

After you have done these four steps you will be able to get the majority of your senses involved whilst you are visualising. I would recommend visualisation for fifteen minutes per day and also that you go through each sense specifically, picturing the sensations felt for each one.

Goal: _____

_____

_____

Sense 1: _____

_____

_____

_____

Sense 2: _____

_____

_____

_____

Sense 3: _____

_____

_____

_____

Sense 4: _____

_____

_____

_____

Exercise: the Cinema Technique

Close your eyes and imagine you are on your own in the cinema. Step out of your body, float up and look down on yourself from a bird's-eye view now watching the film. Onscreen is a black and white film about your ideal life. Now imagine what your ideal life is like or how you want it to be. Who is in your life? Do you have a husband/wife? Do you have children? What do you look like? What do they look like?

Then look more deeply into your own character. How do you stand/talk/walk? How are you dressed? How do your husband/wife and children behave? What are they like? What type of car do you drive and what type of house do you live in? What job are you in, or are you self-employed or a business owner?

Now turn your black and white picture into colour. What colour is your car? What colour is your house? How do others perceive you? Do you have lots of friends? Go further into the details of your life and get extremely specific.

Now imagine you come back down into your body, feeling present and centred.

This could take you five to ten minutes and I would encourage you to do it once a week, or even once a day, depending on how in touch with your goal you want to be.

By performing this exercise you have done something very powerful. You're bringing your goal into the forefront of your mind whilst anchoring it in your subconscious, thus making achieving goals a more efficient process.

Through this technique of visualisation you will be able to incorporate this ideal version of your life into your own. You will begin to walk, talk and act like the man/woman in your film. You will be motivated to be, and will slowly become, the person from your ideal life.

A day in the life

If you could live your life as if you had already achieved your goal, what would it be like? A potential exercise you could do would be to take one random day off work and spend it the way you would if your life was as you had visualised. This is a deeper way to visualise the achievement of your goal, as you are behaving and feeling exactly what it would be like.

This was a particular exercise I found very useful whilst employed. I would take a day off midweek and spend it how I envisioned my life would be. I would get up in the morning, hit the gym, trade whilst in a coffee shop and work on my businesses, which at that point were just at the idea stage. I found this a very helpful exercise as it confirmed to me that this was really what I wanted to do with my life and solidified the goal. I remember thinking to myself 'if I had this much time free every day, imagine what I could achieve in one week, let alone one year'.

'If you can see it in your mind, you can hold it in your hand.'
- Bob Proctor

15. Reflection – the Vital Bonus Step

Although not an actual step in the goal setting process, reflection is key when tracking how far you have come to achieving your goals. This is something I have been doing for years and I have found it very helpful in keeping me focused and on track with my goals. I've personally found that reflections have been very helpful when looking back on the goals I have set.

What is self-reflection?

Self-reflection is like looking into a mirror and describing what you see. It is a way of assessing yourself, your ways of working, and your ways of progression, and this helps you identify what you could improve on in the future.

Why is self-reflection a key?

Reflecting helps you to review the development of your skills. It helps you figure out if you have stuck to your original plan and how you can make sure you continue to do so for the coming months, or begin to do so if you haven't already. In any role, whether at home or at work, reflection is an important part of learning. You wouldn't use a recipe a second time around if the dish didn't work the first time, would you? You would either scrap it or you would alter the recipe until you have the right ingredients to create something special.

Reflective questions you can ask yourself:

Strengths – What are my strengths? For example, am I good at leading? Am I punctual?

89

Weaknesses – What are my weaknesses? For example, do I lack focus? Am I always late for appointments?
Skills – What skills do I have and what am I good at? Am I good at organisation?
Problems – What problems are there in my life right now, whether they be home- or work-related, that I can work on right now?
Achievements – What have I achieved in the last month? Have I created two sources of income? Have I graduated university?
Happiness – Are there things that I am unhappy with or disappointed about? Are there things that have made me really happy? For example: weight, freedom, creating business.
Solutions – How can I improve these areas of my life and what can I do now to work towards that?

Self-reflection can be difficult because it requires you being honest with yourself, which a lot of people don't like to do. But the more you do it, the easier it will be to get honest with yourself. This is self awareness and it can be the fastest way to admit to yourself what you need to do or how to change in order to get closer to your goals and if that requires cutting off poisonous friends or negative people in your life or reducing your time with those people. Would you rather waste years not getting where you want to be because you don't want to hurt people's feelings? It's only going to leave you with the feeling of regret in the future. Reflection isn't just about looking back – it's also there to show you how to look forward, with an end result of giving you more clarity in your life and feeling happier overall.

Exercise: Goal-specific reflective questions

When reflecting on the goals I have set, I find that asking myself the following questions helps me keep on track. Go back and pick each goal you have fully set in turn, and use these questions weekly/monthly/quarterly, or however frequently you wish, to see if you have kept yourself on track.

Goal: _____

_____

Question: What have I done since my last reflection that has pushed me closer to achieving my goal?

1. _____

_____

2. _____

_____

3. _____

_____

4. _____

_____

5. _____

_____

Question: Have I encountered any hurdles since my last reflection? If so, what were they?

1. _____

_____

2. _____

_____

3. _____

_____

4. _____

_____

5. _____

_____

Question: How did I overcome this hurdle?

1. _____

_____

2. _____

_____

3. _____

_____

4. _____

_____

5. _____

_____

Question: How much closer am I to my goal?

_____

_____

_____

_____

_____

Question: What can I do this month that will further push me in the right direction?

1. _____

_____

2. _____

_____

3. _____

_____

4. _____

_____

5. _____

_____

Example: Shaun loves business and fitness, and his goal is to own and run his own gym. He set his goal a month ago and wants to look back on what he has done over the past month to project himself towards it. He has already fully written out his goal in detail, and has read over it before completing this task. It's now time to check in with himself to see how far he has come.

Goal: *I own and run my own gym on or before 31 December 2017*

Question: What have I done since my last reflection that has pushed me closer to achieving my goal?

1. *I have enrolled on a personal training course to increase my knowledge about fitness and learn the techniques required to train others.*
2. *I have written up a full business plan with budgets and savings targets for the next twelve months to ensure I have the capital to lease the building; this includes an average of all monthly outgoings including lease of machines.*

Question: Have I encountered any hurdles since my last reflection? If so, what were they?

1. *The property that I was initially hoping would be available will not be out of lease until March 2019.*
2. *One of the investors has pulled out for personal reasons and I now need to raise more funds.*

Question: How did I overcome this hurdle?

1. *I have researched other buildings in the same area in order to find other potential buildings.*
2. *I have attended an event where the main goal was to bring start-ups and potential investors together.*

> ## Question: How much closer am I to my goal?
>
> *So far I have ticked off fifteen out of a hundred of the manageable steps on my way to achieving my goal. Therefore, I am 15% of the way through and I am seriously motivated to continue to tick off more. My target is to achieve this goal within the next six months and if I continue to tick off fifteen tasks per month it will take me 6.7 months to achieve my goal. Therefore I am on track.*
>
> Question: What can I do this month that will further push me in the right direction?
>
> 1. *I will structure my day more effectively so that I am more efficient with my time and can complete more tasks within the next month.*
> 2. *I will work on more effective ways to market the gym to reach a wider audience, such as emailing a collection of those who may be interested in joining on launch.*

I have provided two examples for each of the goal-specific reflection questions but I would recommend more as this will further push you on your way to achieving your goal, and will keep you focused and on track. You can see from this example how ticking off the small manageable steps can help to motivate and drive you on your way to reaching your goal, Most people don't realise this and are surprised by how much further on they are when they simply reflect on the past weeks and months. Ticking off your manageable steps day-by-day and week-by-week and reviewing them regularly ensures you remain on track. By checking in with yourself monthly and seeing how far you have already come, it can make the initial goal seem less daunting.

I, personally, reflect at the end of each month as I feel this gives me a substantial amount of time to really smash out those manageable steps and I can see a greater progression in the number of them that have been ticked off. This leads to twelve reflections that I can review fully at the end of the year to see how far I have come over the year as a whole. This is a great personal achievement to be able to see all the things you have ticked off each month. Think five year as a whole. This is a great personal achievement to be able to see all the things you have ticked off each month. Think five years down the line when you will have sixty reflections that you can look at and see how much you have grown.

The Twelve Reflections

Imagine having twelve reflections for the whole year to look back on and read how you felt in those moments. Some of the moments may be certain months in which you had a breakthrough or achieved one of your major goals. The important thing here is looking back and reading your reflections from January to December. It is truly an amazing feeling seeing how far you have come and a written story of a year of your life, maybe even a successful formula to share with family members and your kids later down the line. This holds more of a sentimental value but is still also a very important part of your journey. This is why I encourage you to do at least twelve reflections a year, one at the end of every month, to see how far you have come.

'Without deep reflection, one knows from daily life that one exists for other people.'
- Albert Einstein

16. Core Values and Daily Goals

On a subconscious level we already have sets of values, whether we are aware of them or not, that we follow in life.

> Example: Shaun likes to donate regularly to charity and to help children in need. It is very likely that one of the values he holds highly will be giving. This might seem very obvious but sometimes we spend a lifetime trying to work out who we really are when it's actually quite simple.

I have found it helpful to write down a list of five values that are most important to me every day alongside my daily goals. Let me show you.

- Honesty - I am always honest with myself and others and expect the same back from my family, social circle and friends.
- Persistent - I am persistent with the tasks at hand to bring me closer to my goals,
- Passionate - I am passionate about my goals and love what I am working on.
- Caring - I care about my family, friends and myself deeply.
- Laser-focused - I am not just focused but laser-focused, with absolute precision, on goals.

I write down my values every day as a reminder that they are aligned with my goals. It makes you realise that you are working on the goals that are most important to you.

I spent nearly two years working on goals that I thought were really important to me and I don't regret them for one minute as they have shaped who I am today, and I am truly grateful to be able to understand what I really want out of life.

I want you to make sure that you are being true to yourself, as time is precious and should not be wasted on goals that you think you should be working towards from either social or family pressures. It will not make you happy and will leave you feeling unfulfilled. Identifying your core values is singlehandedly one of the most important things you can do because the biggest frustration is working on goals that you think you should be achieving, which are not in alignment with your core values.

If you come to a hurdle and give up on your goal easily you'll find yourself saying 'why can't I follow things through?' or 'that goal was just too hard for me and I need to set more REALISTIC targets'. This is usually to make yourself feel better and to justify why you haven't achieved the goal, when in fact the reason you haven't is because the goal was not in alignment with your core values. We all know what realistic thinking will get you... realistic results, and that's not what we want. You can read about this in more detail in my Smart Goals section.

You have to dig deep, be honest with yourself and ask the question 'if I had no one to impress, or no one to show what I have done, would the goals I am currently working towards really be my goals?' For example, if your goal was to own a Ferrari, but you lived in the most remote of locations and no one would be around to see it, would you still want the Ferrari? Would you want the Ferrari for yourself, or for the impression it gives others of you? I know this may seem like a strange way to think, but sometimes it is the only way to be honest with yourself. I promise you that once you figure out what your core values really are, and then align them with your goals, you'll find that not only is it more enjoyable but hurdles in your way will not faze you, as it will not be a matter of 'if' you achieve your goals but 'when', and any hurdle will just be a minor setback. I find myself smiling when I get a setback because I know I'm on the right path. It gives you the extra support and motivation to keep you focused when you are aware of what truly means the most to you. Sometimes no one will support you or believe in your idea but all you need is to believe in yourself and that's really all that matters.

List of values to help you pick which are most important to you

Happiness	Success	Balance
Wealth	Loyalty	Health
Education	Adventure	Knowledge
Personal Development	Community	Affection
Stability	Power	Culture
Relationships	Respect	Peace
Communication	Love	Fun
Family	Integrity	Growth
Change	Trust	Teaching
Travel	Motivation	Inspiration

From the list I have provided, or from your own values, select five values that most relate to you; the ones that stick out to you are most likely the most important values to you as a person. It is always good to remind ourselves exactly why we are striving for a certain goal. One of the main headaches is not hitting a goal and feeling frustrated by this. This is because it is almost certain that you've been chasing a goal that's not very important to you at that given time in your life. I'm not saying it will never be important to you, but right now it's not.

Now with your values in mind, think about what being successful really means to you. Understanding how you define success means you are able to better succeed in turning your dreams into goals and then into reality. Success to you could mean anything from having a happy family, to being financially secure, to being healthy and fit. Whatever it is to you, write down those answers in bullet points in your journal.

Exercise 1 – Daily Goals

Write down five goals to achieve every day. Start by putting the date at the top followed by your signature, and then your signature again at the bottom right corner of the page.

The reason behind this is because when you sign a document, there is a feeling of obligation to fulfil what you have signed. This will have the same effect on you as when you sign your daily goals; you will feel committed.

Five small goals could be as follows.
- go to the gym – push and pull workout
- one hour of reading/audio book
- thirty minutes road running
- one hour writing out your goals
- meditate for ten minutes using the Headspace app

Tick these goals off as the day goes by and watch the magic happen. When you become accustomed to ticking off these small goals, your mind starts to think 'if I can achieve these, what else can I achieve?"

I like to call this process the conditioning process. You are getting your mind ready – essentially building the mental foundations – for achieving bigger goals! Once you get used to achieving the small goals, tackling the bigger goals seems much easier!

Exercise 2 – Daily Values

Write down your daily goals and then list your daily values. Align your values with your goals. This exercise is designed to help you break through what's holding you back and to put you in line with your goal setting.

Exercise 3 – Affirmations and Signature

After you have listed your goals and values and aligned them with each other, write out affirmations that are going to motivate you to achieve your goals and that are in line with your core values.

Example: Shaun likes to keep fit. Therefore the following could be an example of his three combined exercises.

Daily Goals:
1. Five-mile run in the morning
2. Spend one hour working on new blog post
3. Spend one hour writing out my fitness goal in full using the 10 Steps formula
4. Go to the gym – push and pull workout
5. Spend one hour reading

Values:
1. Integrity
2. Persistence
3. Passion
4. Health
5. Knowledge

Affirmations:
I persist until I succeed.
I persist until I succeed.
I persist until I succeed.
I persist until I succeed.
I persist until I succeed.

Eating only healthy, nutritious, good food is my lifestyle.
Eating only healthy, nutritious, good food is my lifestyle.
Eating only healthy, nutritious, good food is my lifestyle.
Eating only healthy, nutritious, good food is my lifestyle.
Eating only healthy, nutritious, good food is my lifestyle.

Every goal I strive for I do with passion.
Every goal I strive for I do with passion.
Every goal I strive for I do with passion.
Every goal I strive for I do with passion.
Every goal I strive for I do with passion.

> I am 10% body fat with lean muscle on or before 31 Dec 2017.
> I am 10% body fat with lean muscle on or before 31 Dec 2017.
> I am 10% body fat with lean muscle on or before 31 Dec 2017.
> I am 10% body fat with lean muscle on or before 31 Dec 2017.
> I am 10% body fat with lean muscle on or before 31 Dec 2017.
>
> I am laser-focused each and every day.
> I am laser-focused each and every day.
> I am laser-focused each and every day.
> I am laser-focused each and every day.
> I am laser-focused each and every day.

I call this the 555 rule. Your mental 5-a-day. Nutrition for the mind.

Signature – It is important to sign the page each and every day when doing your daily goals, in the same way you would when you are writing out your longer term goals in full as mentioned previously. This ensures that you feel committed.

Prioritisation

If you are the sort of person who finds it difficult to get things done in a way so that the most important tasks are done first, I highly recommend you use colours to trigger your eyes towards your most important daily goals.

Beside your goals put a small circle/box and fill it with the colour it corresponds with. Ensure that the most important boxes are ticked off first.

Red – high priority, must be done, critical
Orange – moderate priority, needs to be done
Green – low priority, to do but still have time to do it after today

Exercise sheet:
GOALS, VALUES AND AFFIRMATIONS

Date:_____

Daily Goals
1._____

2._____

3._____

4._____

5._____

Daily Values
1._____

2._____

3._____

4._____

5._____

Affirmation 1:

_____

_____

_____

_____

Affirmation 2:

Affirmation 3:

Affirmation 4:

Affirmation 5:

_____

_____

_____

_____

_____

Bonus Exercise:

To ensure that your goals are really aligned with your values, you can use this sheet to do so.

Daily Goals
1._____

2._____

3._____

4._____

5._____

Daily Values
1._____

2._____

3._____

4._____

5._____

Link – here you should write the reasons why your values and goals are aligned.

Goal _____ links to Value _____ because_____

_____

Goal _____ links to Value _____ because_____

_____

Goal _____ links to Value _____ because_____

_____

Goal _____ links to Value _____ because_____

_____

Goal _____ links to Value _____ because_____

_____

Goal _____ links to Value _____ because_____

_____

Goal _____ links to Value _____ because_____

_____

Goal _____ links to Value _____ because_____

_____

Goal _____ links to Value _____ because_____

_____

Goal _____ links to Value _____ because_____

_____

There could be a particular goal that links to three different values, or one value that links to multiple goals. Fill in as many as possible. This is not an everyday exercise; do it only when you feel that you need to confirm to yourself why you are working towards a particular goal. This will help you to prove to yourself that it is something you really want as it aligns with your values. Even when this gets tough, it is important to dig deep as that is where new thought patterns begin.

Example: Shaun

Goal 1 links to Value 4 because in order to achieve the goal of running every morning, I'll value health.

For this example (Goal 1) Shaun could have chosen persistence, as this value is also aligned with running. This shows how many goals and values will interlink in many ways. There will not be just one value that links to a particular goal and vice versa.

'Values are like fingerprints, nobody's are the same, but you leave them all over everything you do.'
- Elvis Presley

17. Ten Things I Want to Do, Be and Have

When thinking about goals, it is very common for people to focus mainly on materialistic ones: for example, a specific car they want to own, or perhaps an expensive watch. This is natural, but you need to consider what you need to do and who you need to be in order to achieve many of these goals. In this section I want you all to dig really deep in your thoughts to figure out what you truly want. Through experience I have found that a good way to filter out what you truly want is to list ten things you want to do, be and have.
For example:

'Do' -   To climb a mountain
'Be' -   To be confident at public speaking
'Have' -   To have a red Ferrari

You'll come up with thirty goals in total for the next twelve months that you will focus on achieving. You may begin to write things down and struggle to complete all ten. You may also write down more than ten and realise that some mean more to you than others. It is best to firstly consider everything you would want to do, be and have by the end of the next year, and then to reduce them down (if you have written more than ten for each area) to the thirty that are most important to you. This will not be an easy, simple or quick process. It may take you a couple of days of returning to it to fully complete the ten things for each area.

Do

One of the main reasons that people set goals to 'do' certain things is to feel a sense of fulfilment. Sometimes money is not a big enough incentive and you may need to do things that help you grow as a person. You can have all the material possessions in the world, but if you have not done anything to make yourself feel fulfilled then you can still feel completely empty and unsatisfied. The novelty of material possessions can wear off very quickly, but you cannot buy back the time to do things.

Be

The most motivating part of setting goals to become a certain way is that you are aiming to become the best version of yourself. For many it is easy to pick out parts of themselves that they would like to enhance, improve and change, but if you were to imagine yourself in six months' time, who would you be? Not just appearance-wise, but regarding personality as well as all the other aspects of your being.

Have

These are your material desires. They are natural and perfectly okay. They are your passions and the rewards for your hard work.

Who, what, when, where, how

Who – You.
What – Figuring out if the goals you think are important to you are actually important to you. When you start writing out your goals, you will most likely write the first three to four of each part very quickly and then have to stop and think harder and much more deeply about the rest. You may even find that after getting to ten goals for each, sometimes you cross some out and think of new ones. I like to call this the filtering process.
When – It is best to do this at the beginning of the year but of course you can start whenever you please.
Where – Anywhere: all you need is your journal and a pen.
How – It's simple, if you use the process below.

10 Steps to Achieving Your Goals

<u>Do</u>
1. _____

   _____

2. _____

   _____

3. _____

   _____

4. _____

   _____

5. _____

   _____

6. _____

   _____

7. _____

   _____

8. _____

   _____

9. _____

   _____

10. _____

   _____

<u>Be</u>

1. _____

_____

2. _____

_____

3. _____

_____

4. _____

_____

5. _____

_____

6. _____

_____

7. _____

_____

8. _____

_____

9. _____

_____

10. _____

_____

Have

1. _____

   _____

2. _____

   _____

3. _____

   _____

4. _____

   _____

5. _____

   _____

6. _____

   _____

7. _____

   _____

8. _____

   _____

9. _____

   _____

10. _____

    _____

'The ultimate reason for setting goals is to entice you to become the person it takes to achieve them.'
- Jim Rohn

18. How to Create the Ultimate Vision Board

Many people underestimate the power of a vision board in achieving their goals. But having something to physically look at on a daily basis as a reminder of what you are working towards can be such a strong motivational force.

First things first. Print off a picture of whatever your goal is, be it a house or a car or anything else, on photographic paper. The reason behind this is that standard paper will not make the goal appear as realistic for one particular reason; the whole point of goal setting is to be able to get your mind to believe that you have already achieved the goal before it has happened, so what better way than to have the pictures on your vision board appear to be photos, as photos trigger memories that tell your mind it's real.

This by no means implies that you can just stick a picture onto a board and it will happen. Of course you are going to have to work for it and towards it. This process of printing your goal out onto photographic paper needs to be accompanied by some serious action.

A goal of mine has always been to own a Lamborghini and so I hired one for a week to really experience what it was like to own it. Whilst I did this I took as many photos as I could and pinned many to my goals board. On the back of the photos I have written the date by which I want to have achieved the goal and have signed them, psychologically committing myself to this goal. Remember: 'A dream with a date becomes a goal'. It is difficult to put into words the feeling of having a clearly written out goal with a vision board prepared. The best way to experience it is to do it yourself. Make something to be proud of! Make something that will make you wake up every day and say 'YES! These are my goals and I am doing everything in my power to achieve them.'

Sometimes you just need a boost. It is highly unlikely that a person is positive and feeling the most driven they can be every single day; at the end of the day we are human. We suffer rejections and setbacks and these can leave us feeling deflated and demotivated – but sometimes so do the most successful people in the world. When you look at someone who is successful and think that every morning they wake up with a big smile and full of energy, this is a fantasy and it is best to accept that now. Social media has been a massive player in this game of trapping people into thinking that the lives of the rich and successful are plain sailing and easy going. They have bad days too – stressful days and bad experiences – but that is the part you don't see. We are shown only the fancy watches, big houses and sports cars, not the small bite-size chunks that people take in order to achieve their goals.

In reality, all goals are just bite-size chunks taken consistently. 'Water wears the marble.' This ultimate vision board is designed to keep you on track when you get a setback or get pulled off track.

Step-by-step guide

Here are the simple steps to follow to create the ultimate vision board.

STEP 1: Filter and write out your key goals using the 10 Steps method in your personal journal.

STEP 2: Find/create/buy a vision board. This could be a pin board or white board that you can stick your pictures to as your reminder of what you are aiming to achieve.

STEP 3: Find images that are most applicable to your goal, preferably those that are personal to you. For example, if one of your goals is to own a particular car, rather than just getting an image from the internet, head to the dealer and get a picture of you in the car you want. Seeing yourself already sitting in the car is far more powerful than seeing a picture of a car you found online.

STEP 4: Print your pictures out on photo paper rather than normal paper, as previously mentioned, because this is a signal to your mind of a memory, as if it has already happened.

STEP 5: Sign and date the photograph. This will signal to your brain that you are now obligated to achieve this goal as it will symbolise a contract.

STEP 6: Pin them all onto your vision board to create a collage of all the goals that are most important to you. This will be a constant daily reminder of the hard work you are putting in and of exactly what you are working towards.

STEP 7: Admire daily.

Creating a vision board is actually very simple. Following these steps, you are going to have your own tailored and personal, ultimate vision board that is going to push you towards your goals and remind you daily of what your hard work will result in.

'*Create the highest, grandest vision possible for your life, because you become what you believe.*'
- Oprah Winfrey

19. Summary

Step 1: Set a date – When setting goals it is important to have a set date in mind to spur you on, to give you the extra push you need and to keep you on track. Getting closer to your deadline and knowing you've only given yourself an allocated amount of time will keep you focused. Remember: there are no unrealistic goals, only unrealistic deadlines.

Step 2: Detail is key – Knowing exactly what you want, and writing it out in detail, will be a motivational push for anyone on their way to getting there. There is a big difference between saying 'my goal is to buy a new car' and 'my goal is to own a 2017 Audi R8 that is red with black wheels…' etc. Remember: sign your goals. This will make you feel committed to them, as if you have signed a contract.

Step 3: Manageable steps – Break down your goal into bite-size chunks. You cannot climb a mountain without taking individual steps. This can help to stop your goals feeling so daunting. A big goal can feel intimidating at first, but breaking it down into manageable pieces can make it seem more attainable. Remember: there needs to be an equilibrium between breaking the steps down too much or too little.

Step 4: Identify skills and knowledge required – Could you play in an orchestra without first having learned to play an instrument? This applies to every goal. There will be set knowledge and skills that are needed to help you on your way to achieving your goal. Once you have identified them and begun to work on them, you are one step closer. Remember: a great way to find out the skills and knowledge required is to assess those of your mentors.

Step 5: Identify your obstacles – Identifying what your potential hurdles are at the beginning can make it easier to overcome them. It will stop you feeling so deflated when you come across one, will keep you on track and will keep up your momentum. Hurdles can be frustrating, but they can be overcome and you can continue on your path to achieving your goal. Remember: in reality, you are your only true obstacle.

Step 6: People to associate with – You become an accumulation of the five people who occupy the most of your time. Look out for the red flags in people who will not further you on your journey to achieving your goals, and surround yourself with those who will. 'If you surround yourself with clowns, don't be surprised when your life resembles the circus' (Dr Steve Maraboli). Remember: a giver who gives too much will be left with empty pockets.

Step 7: What is in it for you and why? – Knowing why you want to achieve your goals gives you more purpose. Your why will be your foundation to continue to push you forward. You also need to work out what's in it for you. Trying to achieve a goal because you want to impress someone else or make them happy will not be a strong enough push to get there. You need to know exactly what achieving this goal will do for you. Remember: your whys need to be bigger than the hurdles you may face, otherwise you will not overcome them.

Step 8: What are you prepared to give up? – Everyone is happy to talk about what they want but no one likes to think about what they have to give up to get there. Everything you want you can get if you want it badly enough, as long as you are prepared to sacrifice to achieve your goals. Remember: the biggest rewards come from the greatest sacrifices.

Step 9: Affirmations – The way you talk to yourself and what you say to yourself are highly powerful tools on the path to achieving your goals. Negative self-talk will only lead to pessimism and you will continue to fall short of achieving your goals. Specific, positive language will guide you to the correct way to affirm who you are, and will influence your personality and attitude, which will aid you on your journey to success. Remember: it is highly important to make the affirmations you state closely linked to your goals.

Step 10: Visualisation – Get your senses involved. The aim here is to get your body engaged with your goal setting alongside your mind. Get present: make your goals feel as if they are being achieved right now or have already been achieved. Remember: get as many of your senses involved as possible.

Reflection – the Vital Bonus Step – Reflection is key. It is amazing how motivating it can be to see how far you have come on your way to achieving your goals. If you feel as if you are still so far from them, you can reflect on what you have done in the past to get to where you are now. It also is a driving force in setting new goals as you can reflect on the previous goals you have already achieved, and can see what to do differently when moving forward. Remember: the only time we look back is to see how far we have come.

Evolving goals and rebalancing

Most people get discouraged if they set a goal and do not hit it on the exact date they desire. Although I agree that you should work towards the date as closely as possible, it is also extremely important to acknowledge that when you get taken off track you must rebalance yourself and keep moving forward. Take comfort in knowing that people have achieved some of the greatest goals after countless setbacks. Sometimes your goals may even evolve. Be prepared and open-minded regarding this, as sometimes your goals can grow into something bigger than what you first anticipated. Having a goal that is inflexible could lead to you giving up. But by understanding these principles you will remain positive throughout your journey.

You now have all the steps you need to keep yourself focused and on the path to achieving your goals. You have learned about how positive self-talk can influence your ability to achieve your goals and how you need to interlink your goals into most of the areas of your life. Fed up with your job and want to set up a business? Remember, the wages you are earning can help you to build the capital you need. The values you hold will impact on the goals that are most important to you and that you will therefore be more likely to achieve more quickly.

Whether you have monetary, entrepreneurial, physical, spiritual or any other kind of goals, the 10 steps can guide you on your way to achieving any goal you set your mind to.

'The greatest danger for most of us is not that our aim is too high and we miss it but that it is too low and we reach it.' - Michelangelo

---

Thank you for reading this book. I hope you take away as much value as possible and use it to project you towards achieving any goal you set your mind to. I am a strong believer in a person's ability to accomplish anything that they really want to, and that we are all geniuses, destined for greatness, but sometimes we just need a little guidance to unlock our full potential.

'Allow your passion to become your purpose, and it will someday become your profession.'
- Gabrielle Bernstein

About the author

Mark is a twenty-six-year-old entrepreneur from England. His early years in the world of work were not as successful as he initially hoped. He began training as an engineer at the age of seventeen but was made redundant as the firm collapsed. He then went from job to job, initially working as a labourer and then building himself up to working in positions such as a broker in the City. From a working-class family, Mark has always striven for more, to provide for his family and to build a better life for them all.

He is now the owner of multiple businesses, in areas such as fashion and foreign exchange trading, educating novice through to experienced traders. He began trading forex at the age of eighteen whilst working in his various positions, and now trades fulltime whilst running his companies. Falcon Trading Guidance Limited was his way of teaching others the skills he himself had learned. Passing on his unique style of trading which he has developed since then, he wanted to help others to do what he has, to leave the nine to five of employment and become fulltime forex traders, to have the flexibility and freedom to live the lives they dream of.

Mark found personal development around the same time he was introduced to forex trading and he is passionate about developing his mind as well as his body. He strongly believes in becoming the best version of himself, through continued learning. Goal setting became a great passion of his. He learned quickly that by writing down his goals, and adjusting and developing his formula, he could keep himself focused and continue to work towards his goals with little hesitation. Continually refining his goal setting formula, he came to the realisation that it could help others and not just him. After firstly sharing it with those close to him and seeing how powerfully the changes occurred, he was compelled to share what he had learned and developed with others, empowering them to aim to achieve their goals so that they too could benefit from this formula.

Example Goal

Shaun:

Goal Date: *31 December 2017*

Detail:
I am 10% body fat and very physically fit on or before 31 December 2017. I am lean and muscular. I have broad, round and muscular shoulders, and toned and strong arms. My chest is defined and I have a six-pack showing. I have a noticeable 'sweep' of my quads, defined hamstrings muscles and lifted glutes. My calves are strong and toned. I have a 32 inch waist and a 40 inch chest. I weigh 80 kilograms, which is great for my height of 6ft. I can run a five-minute mile. I resemble the athletic build of a swimmer.

Manageable Steps:
1. *I have set myself four months to lose 8kg of fat, 2kg per month, and build myself a leaner, stronger, more muscular physique.*
2. *I go to the gym five times a week, training each muscle group once as follows:*
   Monday - Back and biceps
   Tuesday - Legs (quad and calves focus) and abdominals
   Wednesday - Shoulders
   Thursday - Chest and triceps
   Friday - Legs (hamstring focus) and abdominals
3. *I train cardio three times a week at the end of my session for thirty minutes, one day of low intensity steady state (LISS) training, one day of high intensity interval training (HIIT) and one day of swimming. This is to ensure that I am burning fat as well as ensuring I maintain muscle.*
   Monday - HIIT
   Wednesday - LISS
   Thursday - Swimming

4. On a Sunday, one of the days off from the gym, I go for a five-kilometre run.

5. I have a macro controlled meal plan that ensures I consume exactly what I need daily to push me closer to achieving my goal physique. Within this I take whey protein powder in my shake straight after the gym to help repair my muscles, as well as fish-oil tablets once a day for my joints and bones and BCAAs during my session for the prevention of lean muscle mass loss. I plan my meals on a Sunday evening and prepare Monday's and Tuesday's food on a Sunday evening, Wednesday's and Thursday's food on a Tuesday evening, and Friday's, Saturday's and Sunday's food on a Thursday evening.

6. On a Saturday evening I allow myself one 'treat' meal where I have any dinner and dessert I wish. This satisfies my craving for foods I know I shouldn't have and therefore keeps me focused throughout the week.

7. I drink three litres of water every day as I am aware of how important it is to keep my body hydrated, especially when training.

8. I take weekly progress pictures on a Sunday and compare them monthly to see my progress.

9. I am aware that there may be interruptions to my gym plan, and that I may not always be able to stick completely to my gym days, but I know there is flexibility in the days I can train as I can always make up missed sessions on Saturdays and Sundays.

Skills and Knowledge required:

1. I am having one session a week with a personal trainer who is teaching me how to remain focused and keeping me on track with my food and progression, as well as pushing me in the intense gym sessions and teaching me the correct form for different exercises. This is something extra to hold me accountable, as I know he will be checking up on my measurements, weight, how much weight I can push/pull and how my fitness is progressing.

2. I am seeking continual advice from a nutritionist to ensure my macro controlled meal plan keeps my body fuelled properly and as healthy as possible.

Obstacles:

1. Fast food - I am focusing on my macro controlled meal plan and living a healthy, sustainable lifestyle.
2. Alcohol - I am aware of the benefits of keeping my body hydrated and therefore I am focusing on these benefits of water on my physiology.
3. Social gatherings - Most restaurants cater for a healthy lifestyle, and therefore when I go out to eat with my friends I ensure I stick to the usual foods I would eat within my meal plan so not to undo any hard work I have put in.

People to associate with:

1. Hardworking, driven individuals such as my colleagues at work
2. Darren, my gym partner, who is on the same fitness journey as I am
3. My personal trainer, who is a fitness enthusiast
4. People striving to achieve goals in general

What's in it for me and why?:

I achieve this goal to have a happy, healthy and long life. What's in it for me is a sustainable lifestyle, where I feel great about myself, have a healthy body, clothes that fit better and feel a sense of achievement. Every time I weigh myself and am closer to my goal weight I am proud; every time I am able to lift more weight or do more repetitions of an exercise I know I have achieved something.

What am I prepared to give up?:

I am prepared to give up foods that do not fit into my meal plan, alcohol as it will not be beneficial to my progress, nights out that may tempt me to cheat on my plan and Friday night movie nights as I am now training in the gym on Friday evenings. I am prepared to give up free/leisure time in order to visit my personal trainer and nutritionist, go to the gym, as well as to prepare and plan my food for the coming week. I will still have time to see my friends/family/partner but I am prepared to give up the appropriate amount of my free/leisure time necessary to achieve this goal.

Affirmations:

I am 10% body fat on or before 31 December 2017.
I am 10% body fat on or before 31 December 2017.
I am 10% body fat on or before 31 December 2017.
I am 10% body fat on or before 31 December 2017.
I am 10% body fat on or before 31 December 2017.

I live a healthy lifestyle.
I live a healthy lifestyle.
I live a healthy lifestyle.
I live a healthy lifestyle.
I live a healthy lifestyle.

I am strong, lean, toned and feel in great shape.
I am strong, lean, toned and feel in great shape.
I am strong, lean, toned and feel in great shape.
I am strong, lean, toned and feel in great shape.
I am strong, lean, toned and feel in great shape.

I always look forward to my workout.
I always look forward to my workout.
I always look forward to my workout.
I always look forward to my workout.
I always look forward to my workout.

I train hard, with intensity in every session.
I train hard, with intensity in every session.
I train hard, with intensity in every session.
I train hard, with intensity in every session.
I train hard, with intensity in every session.

Visualisation:

I am 10% body fat. I see that my clothes fit exactly how I want them to. I feel comfortable and confident. I can see that I have a lean and athletic shape in the mirror and feel great within myself. I see that I look better and hear people pay me regular compliments. I feel positive that I have achieved a lean body that I continually sustain.

Not only is my body lean and athletic looking, but I can see my face is more chiselled and slimmer, and my cheekbones are now more prominent. When running I feel healthy, fast and agile. My friends/family/partner/colleagues look up to me as they see me as a person who is disciplined in achieving goals and can see the progress I have made.

I am on holiday in Mexico. I am lean and in my swim shorts walking towards the sea. I can hear the sounds of the sea, smell salt water, taste the fresh orange juice I have just left beside my sun lounger, feel the sand beneath my feet and sun on my back, and I can look down and see my visible abdominals, muscular legs and lean physique. I feel incredible within myself knowing that I am in great shape, knowing that I have achieved my goal of a lean physique by committing to my plans and staying focused. I know I can achieve any goal I put my mind to with the right steps.

Reflection:

I reflect on my goal every month to see how far I have come.

ONE MONTH LATER...

Reflection:

I am one month into my fitness journey. I have lost 2kg, an inch from my waist and am lifting significantly more weight than I was before. I have cut thirty seconds from my minutes per mile and can already run for longer than before. I am feeling super motivated as I am right on track. I am 25% towards achieving my goal with three months to go. Being on a calorie deficit has made me feel slightly fatigued, but I have been pushing through by keeping my goal in the forefront of my thoughts and seeing the results has pushed me further forward and kept me disciplined. I will keep my focus and look forward to checking in with myself in a month's time to see my improved progress.

Goals

Worksheets

Below are a number of worksheets that can be printed in order to complete the main exercises presented in this book. I usually write my goals in full in a journal but everyone works differently. If you are better off with worksheets, then the following pages will be helpful for you.

Step 1: Set a date

Goal: _____

_____

_____

Deadline:_____

Potential Constraints:

1. _____

_____

2. _____

_____

3. _____

_____

4. _____

_____

5. _____

_____

Step 2: Detail is key

Date:_____

Goal_____

_____

_____

_____

_____

_____

_____

_____

_____

_____

_____

_____

_____

_____

_____

_____

Signature:_____

Step 3: Manageable steps

Goal: _____

_____

Manageable steps:

1. _____

_____

2. _____

_____

3. _____

_____

4. _____

_____

5. _____

_____

6. _____

_____

7. _____

_____

8. _____

_____

Step 4: Identify skills and knowledge required

Possible Mentors:

1. _____   2. _____

3. _____   4. _____

Knowledge questions to ask:

1. _____

_____

2. _____

_____

3. _____

_____

4. _____

_____

Skills questions to ask:

1. _____

_____

2. _____

_____

3. _____

_____

4. _____

_____

Knowledge and Skills:

1. _____

_____

_____

_____

2. _____

_____

_____

_____

3. _____

_____

_____

_____

4. _____

_____

_____

_____

5. _____

_____

_____

_____

6. _____

_____

_____

_____

7. _____

_____

_____

_____

8. _____

_____

_____

_____

9. _____

_____

_____

_____

Step 5: Identify your obstacles

1. Hurdle_____

   Solution_____

2. Hurdle_____

   Solution_____

3. Hurdle_____

   Solution_____

4. Hurdle_____

   Solution_____

5. Hurdle_____

   Solution_____

6. Hurdle_____

   Solution_____

7. Hurdle_____

   Solution_____

Step 6: People to associate with

Person _____

Red Flags: Green Flags:

_____   _____

_____   _____

_____   _____

_____   _____

_____   _____

_____   _____

_____   _____

_____   _____

_____   _____

_____   _____

_____   _____

_____   _____

_____   _____

_____   _____

_____   _____

Step 7: What is in it for you and why?

Why do I want to achieve this goal?

1. _____

_____

2. _____

_____

3. _____

_____

4. _____

_____

5. _____

_____

6. _____

_____

7. _____

_____

8. _____

_____

What is in it for me?

1. _____

_____

2. _____

_____

3. _____

_____

4. _____

_____

5. _____

_____

6. _____

_____

7. _____

_____

8. _____

_____

9. _____

_____

Step 8: What are you prepared to give up?

How I spend my time now (fill in blanks with other time-consuming activities):

	M	T	W	T	F	S	S	Total
Work								
Travel								
Eating								
Sleeping								
Showering and getting ready								
Out with friends								
Out with partner								
Family time								
TV								

How I want to/will now spend my time (fill in blanks with other time-consuming activities):

	M	T	W	T	F	S	S	Total
Work								
Travel								
Eating								
Sleeping								
Showering and getting ready								
Out with friends								
Out with partner								
Family time								
TV								

Step 9: Affirmations

Take one of your goals, and think of two specific and relevant affirmations that apply. Write them out in the correct format and language, keeping them positive and present.

Goal:

_____

Affirmation 1:

1._____

2._____

3._____

4._____

5._____

6._____

7._____

8._____

9._____

10._____

Affirmation 2:

1._____

2._____

3._____

4._____

5._____

6._____

7._____

8._____

9._____

10._____

Affirmation 3:

1._____

2._____

3._____

4._____

5._____

6._____

7._____

8._____

9._____

10._____

Step 10: Visualisation

Take your five senses: sight, touch, taste, sound and smell. Pick four of them (I understand that taste can be difficult to apply to many goals) and choose four ways that you will engage your senses to be able to better visualise your goal.

Goal:

_____

_____

Sense 1: _____

_____

_____

Sense 2: _____

_____

_____

Sense 3: _____

_____

_____

Sense 4: _____

_____

_____

Reflection - the Vital Bonus Step

Go back and pick each goal you have fully set in turn, and use these questions weekly/monthly/quarterly/however frequently you wish to see if you have kept yourself on track.

Goal: _____

_____

_____

Question: What have I done since my last reflection that has pushed me closer to achieving my goal?

1. _____

_____

2. _____

_____

3. _____

_____

4. _____

_____

Question: Have I encountered any hurdles since my last reflection? If so, what were they?

1. _____

_____

2. _____

_____

3. _____

_____

4. _____

_____

Question: How did I overcome this hurdle?

1. _____

_____

2. _____

_____

3. _____

_____

4. _____

_____

Question: How much closer am I to my goal?

_____

_____

_____

_____

_____

_____

Question: What can I do this month that will further push me in the right direction?

1. _____

_____

2. _____

_____

3. _____

_____

4. _____

_____

Core Goals and Daily Values

Date:_____

Daily Goals

1._____

2._____

3._____

4._____

5._____

Daily Values

1._____

2._____

3._____

4._____

5._____

Affirmations

Affirmation 1:

_____

_____

Affirmation 2:

_____

_____

Affirmation 3:

_____

_____

Affirmation 4:

_____

_____

Affirmation 5:

_____

_____

Bonus Exercise:

To ensure that your goals are really aligned with your values, you can use this sheet.

Daily Goals

1._____

2._____

3._____

4._____

5._____

Daily Values

1._____

2._____

3._____

4._____

5._____

Link – here you should write the reasons why your values and goals are aligned.

Goal _____ links to Value _____ because_____

_____

Goal _____ links to Value _____ because_____

_____

Goal ____ links to Value ____ because_____

_____

Goal ____ links to Value ____ because_____

_____

Goal ____ links to Value ____ because_____

_____

Goal ____ links to Value ____ because_____

_____

Goal ____ links to Value ____ because_____

_____

Goal ____ links to Value ____ because_____

_____

Goal ____ links to Value ____ because_____

_____

Goal ____ links to Value ____ because_____

_____

Goal _____ links to Value _____ because_____

_____

Goal _____ links to Value _____ because_____

_____

Goal _____ links to Value _____ because_____

_____

Goal _____ links to Value _____ because_____

_____

Ten Things I Want to Do, Be and Have

Do

1. _____

2. _____

3. _____

4. _____

5. _____

6. _____

7. _____

8. _____

9. _____

10. _____

Be

1. _____

2. _____

3. _____

4. _____

5. _____

6. _____

7. _____

8. _____

9. _____

10. _____

<u>Have</u>

1. _____

2. _____

3. _____

4. _____

5. _____

6. _____

7. _____

8. _____

9. _____

10. _____

The Story of the Falcon and the Crow

Crows can only fly at the heights of tall trees but Falcons can fly thousands of feet in the air. In life, you are going to be surrounded by both Falcons and Crows. Sometimes your goals and ambitions are going to be so big that they seem unobtainable to some people but very achievable to others. The Crows will be those people with limiting beliefs, who think and feel they can only go so far, and only fly so high in life. The Falcons are those who let nothing and no one stand in their way, and who believe that they are capable of anything with the right focus and determination. Falcons are fast, accurate and precise and can see their prey (goal) far in the distance when a Crow cannot.

Now and again, a Crow will look up and see a Falcon flying above them and feel uncomfortable. They will try to bring the Falcon down to their level. The Falcon can adapt and fly lower, at the height of the Crow. But the Crow can never fly at the height of a Falcon.